# Re-Eng

# Trust

*The Missing Ingredient to Fixing Healthcare*

# Jan Berger and Julie Slezak

outskirts
press

"Our whole world is built around the ability to trust"

Unknown

"All of us are driven by the simple belief that the world as it is just won't do-that we have an obligation to fight for the world as it should be"

Michelle Obama

# Table of Contents

# Acknowledgments

This book has been four years in the making. We could have never realized how important the issue of trust would become in our world. The energy for this book has been fueled by our passion to improve healthcare one person and one organization at a time. Julie, you have been a colleague and a friend for over 20 years. Thanks for being my partner in this endeavor and being as passionate in doing our part to improve healthcare. Although Julie and I led the charge in researching and writing this book, it could not have been completed without the support we had from friends and family. I want to thank all of those that completed the surveys and those that trusted us enough to share their thoughts and their stories. In addition, we want to thank the following: Medecision, an organization that understands the importance of trust and for helping with some of the COVID focused research, Susannah Fox for being a cheerleader on those days where the going was slow and tough, Susan Frankle for her support in helping me market the book, Addison Narter-Slezak and Katrina Stadler for helping with the data and research, Molly Moynahan for being a writing coach, advisor and editing the book, and most of all, Julie's husband Dave Narder and my wife, Robin Hochstatter. Not only was Robin a great support by letting me write while she took care of our lives and pushing me when I needed a bit of motivational support, she also helped with the quantitative research and oversaw the ever-growing references portion of the secondary research.

Mom, I look forward to you reading this book. My experiences that helped to shape this book were fueled by you and dad teaching me that speaking up can make a difference.

I want to recognize three other people that helped to make this book possible. All three have since passed away but have left an indelible impact. First is Erwin Levine. He was my professor at Skidmore College that taught me how the past can impact the future. He also taught me that words can change the world. Secondly, is Dr. Robert Gatson. Dr Gatson was my resident advisor at Loyola School of Medicine. Dr Gatson taught me the importance of building relationships with patients, families and colleagues. The third individual, Dr. John McEnery was a private pediatrician that I did moonlighting for during my final year of residency. He believed that the greatest tool a physician has is social cement. These three individuals set a course for me that has led to today's focus on trust.

# Why this book and why now

Healthcare is in the midst of significant change. Some say evolution while others say it is going through revolution. We argue that both are true. The answer lies in what areas of health we are discussing as well as who is being asked. Steven, a parent of three, when asked this question, answered that we are going through a revolution. Steven lost two siblings to cystic fibrosis, a disease that previously killed many individuals as infants or children. Today new medications and surgeries that were unavailable until the last few years are changing lives. On the other hand, if you ask Shannon, a healthcare executive at an urban hospital that continues to focus on the fee for service model of payment with limited value-based contracts, told us that healthcare is always evolving with slow change. His hospital remains focused on the given volume of care within his hospital. "I am not saying that we do not care about quality and value, we do. The reality is the metrics that we spend the most time on is bed days and revenue. We talk about the issue of hospital readmissions, but it is not where we spend our time or energy."

Yes, there are changes occurring in diagnosis, treatment, technology, organizational, operational, and financial models however, the one thing that has remained the same is the importance of trust across healthcare. In fact, we would argue that without trust, these changes whether evolutionary or revolutionary will fail to make an impact. When Julie and I began to discuss the potential for this book two years ago, there was little talk about the issue of trust. David Shore, an educator and author at Harvard University wrote two books on the topic over 10 years ago. Since that time there had been little attention on the topic. As two healthcare executives that had spent the last thirty years in various stakeholder roles within the healthcare ecosystem, we both had become passionate about the topic. The more we spoke with people the more we were convinced that despite the innovation and the changes being made the impact on health and healthcare will be minimal without an honest conversation about the issue of trust.

The words that you will read in this book are not just ours. Yes, we have done a significant amount of primary research. Our words and thoughts are a culmination of our research, as well as secondary research conducted by us and others. Most importantly, we are the carrier of the words and thoughts of the 2000 individuals that have responded to our surveys and 150 individuals that were kind enough to let us interview them on the issue of trust in healthcare. These individuals represent stakeholders across the healthcare environment. Each of them has been willing to honestly share their role in both the degradation as well as the building of trust within one of the largest industries in the U.S.

Julie and I believe that this book is focused on the MOST important factor in health and healthcare today. Trust is THE foundational factor in a highly functional healthcare system

## IN THE GARDEN OF CRISIS, CHANGE BLOOMS

### Words Matter

As the world of health transitions, the healthcare field faces a number of challenges. Some of these changes have caused "wording" or "labeling" challenges. In writing this book, Julie and I found a number of these wording issues. We apologize in advance for those that disagree with our wording choices. There are three areas that we would like to specifically address here.

1. Health versus healthcare. Traditionally, we have thought of healthcare as the formal clinical environment where we receive care. Over the last 20 years we have seen the healthcare world transition from formal "sick" care to one that looks to the broader vision of health. This broader view not only looks at preventative care and social determinants that can affect our health and well -being but also have broadened our view of those that can support our journey of health.

   We have chosen wherever possible to use the word "health" over "healthcare" as health is a broader and more "encompassing" word. We have used the term healthcare when we are addressing an acute or chronic healthcare issue but when we are speaking about issues in general, we will use the word health.

2. Consumer, patient, or member. The name of the person receiving health care varies by who is using the term and the topic discussed. Historically, the word "patient" continues to be used by most healthcare providers. Over the last 40 years, this title has broadened due to a number of reasons including the increasing number of stakeholders that interact with the person receiving services as well as the increasing view that this person should be acting as a "consumer" of the goods and services that they are receiving. Jeff Margolis, the CEO of Welltok, has defined the two terms, patient, and consumer, by differentiating between the action that they are involved with. He defines the patient as one receiving care and the consumer as one that is making choices. The conversation around naming nomenclature tends to create significant emotional response.

We would have loved to use the term "partner" in order to better articulate the desired balance of power and responsibility that is evolving, but we have chosen to use the term "consumer" in this book whenever possible as consumers also have a more equilibrated relationship with those that they interact with. In addition, the term "consumer" also speaks to the knowledge, optionality and decision making that is necessary in the health and healthcare environment of this century.

3. Doctor versus provider- Like the term "consumer," the words doctor versus provider creates a significant emotional response. For a large portion of the 20th Century, doctors were perceived as the primary person involved with a patient and their healthcare. This is not to say that nurses, dentists, pharmacists, and many others did not deliver care. It is the reality that the "captain of the ship" in care was most often a physician. In interviewing a number of people regarding the topic of terminology of doctor versus provider, there are those that feel that a provider is one that delivers a commodity and does not respect the skill that a physician offers to the person that they care for. Some physicians feel that utilizing the term "provider" is a reduction in status. The word doctor is over 800 years old and comes from the Latin word "church father." The word physician comes the Latin word physic, or natural science and artist of healing.

In this book we will be using the term "healthcare provider" when we are speaking about any individual that is supporting the health of a consumer. We found that as healthcare has broadened to health, providers have also expanded in both who the individual is as well as what that individual does. By choosing the term "provider" we are not looking to be dismissive or disrespectful to anyone. We will be more specific in terminology if we are discussing a specific type of healthcare provider or retelling a story from our qualitative or quantitative surveys.

# SECTION ONE: THE BASICS

# The Biology of Trust

*As Julie Andrews sings in The Sound of Music;*
*"Let's start at the very beginning."*

Trust is innate. It is what encourages a baby to relax and thrive in an environment, knowing she is safe. Humans are actually hard wired to make social connections through trust. Our biology impacts our ability to trust other humans. Trust is spontaneous initially but not indefinitely. However, we have a propensity towards trust. Society, genetics, and family can all impact trust. Trust can be eroded. Giving and earning trust is an important act. The human brain has two neurological alignments that allow us to trust others both inside and outside of our immediate and intimate relationships. The first is an area called the hypertrophied cortex, which is the area of the brains outer surface. This is the area of the brain that helps us to consider "What would I do if I were in this person's position." It allows us to react in accordance to how we believe other people will act under the circumstances. This reaction has a direct impact on our willingness to trust another. Oxytocin modulates the second area of biological impact on the human brain in regard to our ability to trust, a neurochemical whose receptors are in the frontal cortex of the brain. Oxytocin regulates social behavior in animals including the ability to interact and attach emotionally to others. (Zak, HBR Ascend). Emotional and physical touch creates oxytocin which increases trust.

A 2005 study found that a subset of individuals treated with oxytocin prior to interacting with participants in a gaming situation were more trusting of the other participants than those not treated with oxytocin. (Baumgartner et al., 2008) Although other animals have oxytocin and associated receptors, humans have the most, allowing us to have a reduced level of anxiety when we are interacting with others and to interact and cooperate more than other species. These two areas when working together allow us to answer the questions of "should I trust you, how much do you trust me, and how should I interact with you?" (Haas BW, Ishak A. Anderson I, Filkowski M. The Tendency to Trust is Reflected in Human Brain Structure. Neuroimage, February 15, 2015 107:175-181) A second study, done by the University of Michigan, showed that children display judgement associated with trust at an early age. The researchers worked with 4-6-year-old children to determine how trust impacted their interactions with other children of their age. Rosati and his study partners found that the children in the research study were quite accurate in identifying who was a trusted and untrusted partner. The team found that interpersonal trust develops early in development. (Wadley Jared, Rosati Alexandra, Children learn to trust, invest in others at an early age, University of Michigan News, July 23, 2019)

How does it make you feel when someone reaches out to offer a supportive touch? In most cases, we are more likely to trust that person. This response is due to chemical release from our brains. The 1979 AT&T commercial used the tag line "reach out and touch someone" to articulate the feeling of communication and relationship. It also addressed the human need for relationship and created trust in the brand.

Through biology our bodies create presumptive trust. Our biology also has an impact on whether we trust someone after they have broken our trust. If trust is tested repeatedly through experiences which erode trust, the brain will create a natural instinct that reverses the natural inclination to trust.

## What is Trust

Marge is a healthy 70-year-old woman with the exception of having high cholesterol. She has seen the same physician for years and has been happy with him. Her only medicine lowers her cholesterol. She has been on this medicine for several years. During this time, a generic of her medicine releases on the market. A family member suggests she try this generic. She asks her physician to switch to this generic saving her a great deal of money. Her doctor responds by saying that since she is doing well, there is no reason to change. She again requests the switch promising to follow up in three months to make sure that the new medicine is working. After a blood test proves that Marge's cholesterol is normal, Marge shares her frustration with her doctor saying," if you ever cost me $75 dollars a month unnecessarily again, I will change doctors. I no longer trust you as you clearly do not have my best interest (in mind)."

Several questions arise from Marge's story. What is this "trust" that she is talking about? Does trust matter? Can her physician regain her trust after losing it?" Does her provider care whether he or she has Marge's trust?

George is a nurse that works with Dr Stevens and his medical group. When he returned from active duty in the military, he had a choice of joining several primary care groups. He chose Dr Stevens group because of their reputation of putting the patient first and of doing more than expected. George trusted this group of providers as they would never compromise the values that he had.

George was clear in his trust for Dr Stevens and the other providers in this group even though he had never worked with them. What made George trust this group?

Sam is a benefits executive for a mid-size employer who chooses an insurance company to administer benefits for their employees and their families. Sam uses a healthcare benefits consulting company to aid in the decision-making process. When asked why he utilizes this third party he shared with us that he "needs someone who knows the tricks that insurance providers try to play."

Sam's story adds some additional questions about business relationships; has Sam experienced situations where there is an erosion of trust or is this a pre-emptive action? Is trust important in this type of business transaction?

These are examples of how trust impacts healthcare. Trust is an action and reaction, not just found in the health and healthcare environment but throughout all societies.

> The television show *Cheers* ran from 1982-1993. The setting was a Boston bar where "everyone knows your name." The characters had a relationship and trusted each other. Why do you return to restaurants? Many of us often go to the same restaurant because we enjoy the environment, believe that the food is good, and safe. We trust it so we return.

We will come back to Marge, George and Sam, and the issues associated with trust within the healthcare system later. First, we want to talk about trust in society as a whole.

> "Lions and Tigers and Bears, Oh My." This famous phrase used by the Tin Man, Dorothy and the Scarecrow in T*he Wizard of Oz* expresses their fear of the dark forest and the world they found themselves in. Maneuvering in a world without trust can create a similar sense of fear.

Over the course of this book we will explore how trust and healthcare have a unique and tumultuos relationship. We will use survey and interview results to describe the practice of medicine and the healthcare system through the eyes of each of the stakeholders. Through this journey we hope that our findings will help others to see a path to improving trusting relationships and outcomes associated with our health and healthcare systems.

Confucius stated that rulers need three resources

1. Weapons
2. Food
3. Most important, trust

While trust is a universal ingredient in well- functioning societies, there is disagreement about the meaning of trust. To discuss the definition of trust, let's take a step back and see if we can create a mutual understanding of the word. There has been much conversation over the years that focuses on the role of trust in both personal and professional relationships. We believe that for us to positively influence trust we need to agree on a clarification of trust or at least some interpretation of what trust is.

Unfortunately, there are many definitions associated with trust, similar in some ways but different in others. This makes agreeing on a definition difficult. I ask you to pause a moment and turn to a colleague, friend or family member and ask them to define the word trust. It is hard to define the term. Webster dictionary states that trust is the "assured reliance on the character, ability, strength, or truth of someone or something." (Webster Dictionary). Oxford dictionary states that trust is the "firm belief in the reliability, truth, or ability of someone or something" (Oxford dictionary) The Mosby Dental Dictionary states "relationship in which one person or entity holds fiduciary responsibility for another's property or enterprise."

David Shore, a well-known Harvard Professor, in his book *The Trust Crisis*, stated "trust is the currency of all commerce." Whereas David Thom in his article in Health Affairs defined trust as "social capital" (Health Affairs, David Thom) Thom continued to say that trust is an essential ingredient for all societies, a powerful lubricant that supports interactions to function at their fullest. Nobel Prize Winner Kenneth Arrow stated that things do not work without trust, in fact, without trust in both people and systems, institutions fail. Although these three scholars view trust through slightly different lenses, all three see trust as a key component of all human societies. Trust is a construct based on sociological tenets. It comes from both our head and our hearts. Humans are social animals who need to cooperate in order to survive. If we do not trust each other on some level cooperation is nearly impossible. Trust is essential for all types of relationships. An organized functional society requires trust (Kramer R, Tyler T. Trust in Organizations).

During our interviews we asked the participants to define trust. Many stated that their definition varies depending on the circumstance and situation. We found a number of words or phrases repeated in peoples' definitions including:

- reliability,
- intentionality,
- your interest over theirs,
- acceptance of a vulnerable situation
- how one acts during that vulnerable period,
- one's expectation of competency,
- good will,
- integrity and commitment,
- ability to feel safe when vulnerable,
- predictability,
- a feeling or belief that something will work or that someone will do something,
- trust is a collection of expectations that someone will do what is best for you and put their needs behind yours,
- honesty and vulnerability,
- feeling seen and known,

- the need for interdependency,
- the need for consistency in action,
- trust is the acceptance of a vulnerable situation where the vulnerable party believes that the other party or parties will have the vulnerable persons best interest in mind.

A number of individuals could not agree upon a definition of trust, because trust is so personal.

Samantha, a middle school teacher, was asked to give us her definition of trust. After sitting quietly and pondering the conversation she stated "I don't believe that there is one definition of trust. In fact, if you were to ask me today and then again tomorrow, it is very likely my definition would change. I think that trust is based on an individual's life experiences. I am not even sure that I could give you a consistent answer on what or who I trust. It is such a nuanced feeling and therefore my answer is constantly changing"

Even lacking a consistently agreed upon definition, a few themes frequently arose during these interviews. The first theme is the interaction between trust and relationships. **Trust and relationships** have a "chicken and egg" relationship. In order to have a successful relationship individuals and organizations need to trust each other and in turn, it is difficult to trust someone without first forming some type of relationship. Both trust and relationships form the intimate social networks and framework for our lives and for society. Simon Sinek has written and spoken a great deal about trust. He believes that trust is necessary for the survival of the human race. Others have said it is the lubricant of societal interaction and is woven into everything we do.

Stephan shared with me his confusion about which comes first, the relationship or trust. He stated in some cases it is easy; "I chose a carmaker and bought my car because I trusted it to be reliable, I then built a relationship with the car dealer." He went on to share that the relationship between a personal relationship and trust are not that clear. "I met my college roommate and started a relationship with him. Trust grew out of that relationship. At the same time, I do not think I would have grown to have a relationship with him if I did not trust him to be a reasonable guy."

The second theme focuses on, the role of **vulnerability** in the process of trust. Trust requires a person to be vulnerable, placing their well-being in the hands of another. It requires one to have confidence that the other person or institution will put their own best interest aside in order to take care of them. Trust must be earned. Just because you either know someone or work with them does not mean that there is trust between the individuals.

Lola is a 55-year-old corporate executive offered a promotion into a new division of the organization where she worked. Lola shared that although she had worked hard for the promotion, she chose not to take it because she trusted her present boss while she did not trust her potential replacement. "He was someone who really looked out for himself first, if something went right, he took credit whereas if something went wrong it was never his fault."

The issue of trust and vulnerability is one that will take center stage in our conversations regarding trust within the health and healthcare environment.

The third issue that we want to take a moment to address is the fact that trust is not unit-directional nor passive. Trust does not work if it is not **mutual.**

Sally, during her interview, described how trust works by comparing it to dancing. "It is never as much fun to dance alone. It just doesn't work well. I see trust the same way. Trusting someone that does not trust you is lonely".

Finally, we want to take a moment to clarify the temporal issues associated with trust. Trust includes both the past and the future actions. When we trust someone, we are depending on the future behavior of another person. We are believing that this person has "moral competence," and a concern for our well-being that is going to impact how they behave in the future. Although it is future directed, it is often based on past experience.

Solomon tells the story of the weekly executive team meetings that he attended. The CEO of the company constantly badgered and belittled his direct reports, of which Solomon was one. Solomon held his breath throughout each meeting waiting for the meeting to be over hoping not to be humiliated. Unfortunately, Solomon lost his father during his tenure in this company. When the CEO called him to offer his condolences, Solomon did not return the call.

We think that Bridget Duffy, a well-respected healthcare executive that focuses on the consumer experience within healthcare and the original designer of patient experience leading to trust stated it best; "trust is an investment of time, energy and money. It is also one that gives back in innumerable ways." She goes on to say, "Trust makes healthcare more impactful and fulfilling for everyone."

## Trust in healthcare

"Trust is like oil for a car, it is necessary for the proper functioning (of healthcare)." This statement is from Justin, a three- sector healthcare executive. He has worked in the government, in the provider space and as a corporate healthcare executive. When asked if he thought that his analogy of trust being like oil for a car was any different in healthcare than it is in any other area of society, his answer was yes and no. "It is similar in that in general it is true in any area of society, but healthcare is just more complex, and the impact can be greater because we are talking about a person's life. That is really serious stuff."

As we have shared, trust is the cement that holds the bricks of society together. It is a crucial element for a functioning society. The importance of trust is especially true in healthcare. Along with financial services, nowhere is trust more desired and needed than in healthcare. Interestingly, both our health and our financial wellbeing are basic to our survival. Healthcare is an environment where we are at our most vulnerable and trust counts the most. How a patient engages, is related to the trust they have in their doctor and the system. Trust within the health and the healthcare environment is one of the most complex relationships in society.

We asked many of the people that we surveyed whether they felt that trust in healthcare was different than issues of trust in society as a whole. The answers that we received were fairly consistant. People stated that although there are some similarities between trust in society and trust within healthcare, there are also a number of differences. Alan Spiro in his healthcare blog stated that healthcare is based on a "sacred trust" (Spiro, Healthcare Blog 4/26/15). Dr. Spiro's statement was similar to Crawshaw and his co-authors when they stated that "medicine is a moral enterprise grounded in a covenant of trust." Both of these thoughtful experts spoke to the same issues identified by the survey takers, health and healthcare are extremely personal. Trust is different in healthcare than in other areas of our lives. We are vulnerable when we trust others with our lives.

We spoke with Stan, a 59 year old teacher. During our conversation with Stan, he talked about his belief that the issue of trust is a new phenomena. I asked Stan why he thought that issues of trust were a new issue. He shared " The world is different. It used to be that people just trusted each other because the world was simpler…people were open and honest with each other." When I asked him if this was true in healthcare as well, he shared that " doctors and patients did not have a financial relationship…" This created a world where doctors were open and honest."

Issues of trust have deep historical roots. Trust developed early in human history as a survival skill. People could not survive in a strange setting alone, without the help of others for food and security. Trust not only plays a role in basic survival but also has had a longstanding role in healthcare. For centuries trust was the ingredient that made medical care viable. There were few diagnostic capabilities, and a paucity of medications, surgeries and other forms of intervention and treatment. Early physicians did not think of the relationship between themselves and the patient as one of equality. The patient was expected to be passive and follow the dictates of the physicians. The granted authority was based on their stature or their training and knowledge. This belief dates back to 2600 BC. Imhotep, an Egyptian leader in healthcare and an early father of healthcare was considered a God of medicine. Therefore, those around him trusted this deity to cure them of their ills. The trust came through his status as a God and nothing else. Hippocrates (460 BC-375 BC), the Greek physician that is known by many as the father of medicine had three rules that were necessary for medicine which included:

1. Being well groomed
2. Being kind to patients
3. Maintaining the highest integrity

If you think about these rules, all of them lead to trust. Although Hippocrates was seen as the ideal physician and young physicians entering the field of medicine recited the Hippocratic oath, he felt that doctors should conceal "most things from the patient including the patients present or future conditions." (SF Kurtz) Hippocrates went on to say that it was appropriate to withhold information regarding medical formulas and medication information with patients. Hippocrates believed that a physician does not share information of care specific to a patient or in general with any other person unless they had signed the covenant of the Hippocratic oath. The only people that signed the oath were physicians. Plato another well-known person agreed with Hippocrates in that he felt that "lies for good and noble purposes were fine when doctors were treating patients" (Topol pp19). This lack of transparency of information and inequality of power continued for many centuries.

The issues of trust continued into the future. Isaac Israeli, a foremost physician who lived from 832-932 AD suggested that physicians should refuse to work with difficult patient or those that did not follow his orders. He felt that the energy between the doctor and the patient was" unhealthy" when the patient was not completely trusting of the physician's recommendations (Topol pp19) (Jerusalem Post January 17, 2016).

It was not until the 16th or 17th century that you find that doctors beginning to believe that patients should have a voice in their care, treatment, and cure. This change in belief lasted only a short period of time. In 1847, the American Medical Association (AMA) was formed. As the largest professional organization of physicians in the United States, it has greatly influenced physicians in how doctors felt and acted. The original code of ethics stated that the obedience of a patient to the prescriptions of his physician should be prompt and implicit. The patient should never send for a consulting physician without express consent of his own medical attendant. As one can infer from this code, the patient was to follow the orders of his physician solely. Questions, interchange, and trust were not even considered. If we jump to 1903, the Revision of Principles of Medical Ethics stated, "A solemn duty to avoid all utterances and actions having a tendency to discourse and depress the patient." Informed consent did not come into action until 1957 when a further revision of the Principals stated that physicians were obligated to disclose all facts relevant to the care of a patient." Although this was written in the Principals it was rarely followed. A JAMA article from 1961 found that 88% of physicians had a policy of not telling their patients that they had the diagnosis of cancer. In fact, as recently as the 1980s, physicians were entitled to treat without consent of the patient when the physician believed consent would be medically contraindicated (Topol pp25). The issue of disclosure and transparency of information is not one that has been completely resolved. In 2012, the AMA stated that patients should not have access to their own data including their DNA. Today the controversy remains over whether or not a patient has the right to see their own medical record. Clearly, elements of trust, such as equality and transparency between the physician and the consumer has had a tortured history. In reality, trust like many other trends within healthcare is cyclical and has to be put in context to both internal and external environmental issues.

David Shore stated in his book that "we suffer from a trust famine." (Shore TC) Twelve years later that "famine' has only increased. Was this always the case? The answer in general is no, but it is not an easy question. Our health is a life and death issue. Like life, healthcare, requires different relationships depending on the situation. Each system, whether it be political, economic, or healthcare, requires trust as an essential element. This is even more true in healthcare. Let's go back and re-visit Marge, George, and Sam. All three individuals that we introduced you to at the beginning of the book.

For each of these cases, the basis of trust is different. In the case of Marge, the focus of trust was based on a personal relationship and interaction. Marge felt that her doctor was not focused on her best financial interest. In the case of George, the basis of trust was reputational and not due to an actual personal experience. In the third case, Sam based his trust on the third party's knowledge or competence. Trust is not uni-dimensional there is more than one type of trust and trust resets. We will go into depth on these topics in a bit.

Trust in healthcare is significantly impacted by its external environment and society. Trust in healthcare does not occur in isolation.

The degradation of trust is caused by a mixture of external and internal issues as well as self -inflicted actions and wounds. Conflict, scandal, and bad behavior in society, whether within the healthcare system or outside, impacts on how people see and feel about healthcare.

In 2003 Elizabeth Holmes founded Theranos, a healthcare technology corporation. The corporation valued at $200 billion dollars in 2014, was touted as a company that would revolutionize healthcare by making blood tests less expensive and "patient friendly." In 2015, John Carreyrou of the Wall Street Journal broke a story questioning the validity of both the technology utilized and the company itself. In 2018, the company ceased operations after being sanctioned by CMS and organizations such as Walgreens terminated its contract and sued the organization. The SEC charged both Elizabeth Holmes and Ramesh (Sunny) Balwani with fraud. This story has been told numerous times by the media with articles, books, movies, and TV News segments. The very public scandal around Theranos, along with other unethical healthcare behavior has led to an erosion of trust across the healthcare ecosystem. Gallup during a 2016 survey measuring trust in healthcare, found that an increasing lack of trust in institutions as a whole in society had an impact on the perception of healthcare. Clearly, people do not differentiate healthcare institutions from other types of societal institutions. (Chou, Oh et al).

In addition to the general degradation in trust within the United States, there are several societal trends that have directly impacted trust within healthcare. The first is the increased level of transiency in society. As we will discuss throughout the book, trust is based in most cases on the quality of a relationship. For the most part our relationships do not have their former longevity. That is not to say that there are not geographies within the United States where individuals live their entire lives in the same community. A Pew study in 2009 found that 30% of individuals spent most of their lives within 100 miles of where they were born. When asked why they stated so close to home, many shared that it due to family and community. It was where they felt safe and loved. For the most part, this is not the case. A 2009 survey stated that a large part of those surveyed felt that a major portion of the country was "restless and rootless." The transient nature of society creates a challenge to the issue of trust in general. Regarding one's health and healthcare it is felt even more intensely.

## Decline of Trust in the Medical Community

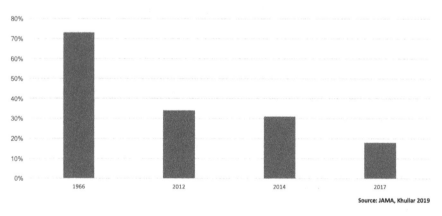

Source: JAMA, Khullar 2019

As you will read throughout the book, type and length of relationship matters in healthcare. Relationships within society as a whole have changed. Toyin Ajayi MD, Chief Health Officer of the organization CityBlock talks about "lazy proxies" for trust instead of true relationships. This is also true within healthcare. It used to be that individuals would have their primary care provider for years, but that relationship is rare now. The reasons for this vary but include:

1. We move more often that we used to. Whether this move is by the consumer or the provider, mobility impacts the length of the relationship
2. Health insurance network rosters are not stagnant. It is not unusual for the consumer to have the same insurance but have different doctors in their network from one year to the next
3. Health insurance for the individual may change. Employers often change their health insurer, and this may impact the ability of the consumer to continue to see their primary care provider.

Interestingly, there is one area that conflicts with the issue of relationships within healthcare, obstetrics, and pediatrics. It is not unusual for a woman (whether they are the one that carries the health insurance, or it is their spouse) to decide which health insurance a family will choose between those offered by following their obstetrician's and/or their children's pediatrician's advice. The bond of trust is strongest or most important when it comes to these two areas.

The third societal trend that directly impacts healthcare is the fact that healthcare has become more organizationally complex and institutionalized. Trust in healthcare has eroded due to confusion, its focus on profits, impersonal interactions, fear and rumor. As healthcare has increased in complexity (cost, science, and treatment), it has created greater complexity in the trust equation.

Trust is no longer an issue solely between the doctor and the consumer, it now includes many other stakeholders. The numbers of people and organizations involved in healthcare has had a direct impact on these metrics associated with trust. Changes in delivery systems, clinician/consumer relationships, payment changes, changes in media, increase in technology, increases in diagnostic and treatment options all impact trust. As we discussed earlier in this chapter, much of healthcare was formerly based in a dyad relationship between the consumer and their doctor. Although there were insurance systems prior to the 1960s, Medicare ushered in an era of increasing stakeholders engaging both directly and indirectly in the healthcare environment. Studies have repeatedly shown that individuals trust institutions less than they trust people. As Stan, who you met earlier, stated "healthcare is now a "thing," it is not about people. It is based on organizations and about organizations. There is no focus on people in healthcare. "I just don't trust things" Stan said. In 1966, three quarters of Americans had confidence in those involved in their healthcare. 73% of those surveyed stated "they felt a great deal of confidence and trust in medicine. Healthcare has not seen that level of trust in the healthcare system since that time. Trust and confidence hit an all-time low in the 1990s with only 20% stating they had confidence in the health system. Fast forward to 2019, and that number drops to 18% (Edelman, David Shore, Trust Crisis, JAMA Khullar 2019) As you can see, scales have ranged between 20-50% since the "heyday" of healthcare trust. The message that we receive is in spite of significant improvements in technology, diagnostics, treatments, and medical outcomes for serious conditions, trust has deteriorated.

The fourth societal trend that has a significant impact on trust within the healthcare ecosystem is the advancement of knowledge. A University of Ottawa article written by Sarah Boon in 2009 stated that there were 2.5 million journal articles published annually. Think about it, this is only the published information. Now consider how much additional information bombards us. The article goes on to talk about the 21st Century Science Overload that we all encounter. It spoke about how people are deluged by new information and facts. (Boon Sarah, 21st Century Science Overload, Canadian Science Journal, January 7, 2017). This issue is even more acute in healthcare. It is believed that there are 80,000 healthcare articles published annually. Again, this is in formal journals and not from other types of formal information sharing such as conferences or the many forms of informal information sharing that take place in today's society. This onslaught of new information in healthcare has placed pressure on trust throughout the industry. One of the challenges to healthcare and trust is the fact that science keeps evolving. This evolution creates conflicts on what we should do in order to keep healthy. Examples include our breakfast; is coffee or eggs good for us, or even safe? Other examples include issues around hormone replacement therapy for women in menopause or the use of low dose aspirin replacement to reduce one's likelihood of a heart attack. This information overload creates both confusion and conflict as well as potential reduction in trust. Earlier in the book we talked about how individuals defined trust. One word that used repeatedly was consistency. Humans crave consistency. When information is inconsistent or conflicting, it tends to reduce our trust in the information as well as reducing our trust in those that are delivering the conflicting information.

Sanjay is a 40-year-old physician. He practices Internal Medicine in an upper middle- class suburban community. Sanjay shared with us his frustration in this fast-moving informational era. "I spend every Sunday afternoon reading medical journals. Even with all the time I spend, I don't feel like I can keep up. To make matters worse, I can read two journal articles that have conflicting information. This is really frustrating." Sanjay went on to share a story from his own practice. For several years Sanjay was advising all his patients over the age of 50 to take low dose aspirin as a preventative means to heart attacks. Fast forward 5 years and now he is telling his patients that not only may this not help but it may put them at risk for a bleeding event. He shared that he had several patients that stated that his conflicting advice made them nervous and therefore they would be finding another physician.

Today, creating trusting relationships both within our society as a whole and in healthcare in general is a challenge. Before we can identify ways to begin healing the "trust famine" (Shore) there are a few areas where we need to delve more deeply. Each of these building blocks will allow us to begin to formulate a plan for healing the trust crisis.

## Types of Trust

Consumers have come to expect trust across all industries and all activities as trust is a global concept. Although trust is a broad overarching idea it does not mean that there is a singular type of trust. As shared previously, there are a number of definitions associated with trust. None of those definitions are definitive. What we find is that there are several typologies and a number of factors that go into trust, in the end it all feeds into the single concept of trust.

It is our belief that trust includes both the head and the heart. Trust in healthcare utilizes both sides of one's brain, the right side for emotional trust and the left side for intellectual trust. We are not alone in this belief. Throughout our interviews we continuously heard people talk about both emotional and empathy-based forms of trust as well as the more credentialed and competency- based attributes of trust. A paper within JAMA talks about the impact of both structure and situation on trust. Structures being agreements made and honored consistently. Situations means there are shared rules and values integrated into interactive processes. (Stout et al). In order for us to discuss how our actions and beliefs impact trust we must identify what definition of trust is best for a specific purpose and under what conditions. Throughout the book, you will see how the distinctive typologies associated with trust come into play within healthcare. There are numerous views of trust and a few methodologies used when discussing trust. We have chosen to present five trust typology methods in this chapter. Each of these methods of looking at trust add a nuanced and unique layer to the interwoven tapestry that makes up trust.

The first method of trust typing breaks down trust between:

1. Competency
2. Character or agency including interpersonal relationship (communication and empathy), agency (fidelity, loyalty, and/ or fiduciary duty, putting the patient first over the clinician's own needs, desires, and best interests)

Let's start with competency and its role in trust. When one talks about competency in terms of trust, they are often speaking about one's physical capability, intellectual knowledge, skill set or ability to perform the task that you need them to perform. Has the individual done this activity before? What was the outcome? Competence leads to credibility and then confidence. Competence allows individuals to overcome fear and vulnerability as well as gain respect. David Shore in his book stated that "patient trust is trust in the clinical skills and knowledge of the physicians, other professionals and service organizations with whom the patient comes in contact with." The association between competence and trust is not only found in healthcare. Think about taking your car for repair. We need to trust that the repair person knows what they are doing. Most of us do not have much knowledge about the inner workings of a car. Therefore, there is a knowledge discordance. Any time we are placed in a position of knowledge discordance, competency trust comes into play. I must trust that the person fixing my car is competent.

Medical competence is often the type of trust we first think of when thinking about trust in healthcare.

Sasha shared with us that when she walks into a physician's office for the first time, she always looks for the doctor's diplomas. To her, the diplomas and documentation of their successful education makes her comfortable that the physician is competent to treat her. When we asked her, what she does if the medical diploma is not on the wall, she stated that she will begin the visit by asking the doctor about where and when they graduated from medical school. Most recently she has begun to do a search on the physician prior to the visit in order to gather this information proactively.

Is the assumption of competency on the part of healthcare providers a form of "blind trust?" Reality is that it is not easy to know whether a doctor is competent. Is the doctor keeping up with the newest care? What if the doctor is competent in one area but incompetent in others? For some consumers, competency can go beyond education.

Robert went to a new doctor. He did not know anything about this doctor except for the fact his insurance that covered this doctor and was affiliated with a hospital system that he trusted. Robert got to the office for the first time. The staff was rude, the office seemed disorganized and the bathroom was dirty. Robert felt that if the doctor did not care about these details that he probably did not care about other details and did not trust his care. Without being seen Robert left the office.

Most of us do not know how to measure the competence of another. It is a perception. People often utilize "substitutes" for competence, as was the case with Robert since he used the support staff's attitude and the lack of cleanliness.

The issue of competence is not relegated solely to the consumer-provider relationship. The issue of competence is often part of the mistrust undercurrent found between healthcare providers and those that focus on the business end of healthcare. We do not have to go any further than one of the co-authors of this book to find an example of this issue.

Jan began her professional carrier as a practicing pediatrician. Not long after beginning her clinical career, Jan realized that she also more enjoyed the business side of medicine. As Jan transitioned into more administrative roles, she repeatedly hit roadblocks from those that believed that "doctors have no business sense." After several frustrating experiences, Jan chose to go back and get an additional degree, hoping to overcome the perception of others. Over time, Jan's experience as a businesswoman overcame this bias and lack of trust in Jan's capabilities as a business executive.

Unfortunately, this prejudice continues today as a significant number of healthcare executives, including hospital and system administrators and health insurance executives have limited trust in someone that has trained as a physician to be an effective healthcare executive.

Fukayama, in his 1996 paper, spoke about the fact that we "trust a doctor not to do us deliberate injury" (Fukayama). What we don't know is whether Fukayama was speaking about a doctor having competence through mastering their craft through education and experience or trusting a doctor to be consistent, reliable, empathetic, and compassionate. These skills or attributes focus on the second type of trust listed above; character and agency. Although competence is important, for most people, one's character and intent are equally important.

Like competence, there is no real test for benevolence, caring, empathy and integrity. As Abraham Lincoln stated, "To ease another's heartache is to forget one's own." Interpersonal skills and compassion often aligned with patient centered care within the Patient Centered Medical Home and Accountable Care Organization programs have recently taken on new importance. One of the foundational beliefs associated with these programs is that the trusting relationship between a consumer and their provider will create a bond that improves outcomes within the system. While we believe in the importance of this type of trusting relationship whether it impacts outcomes in the manner that many people hope is still unclear.

Like the issue of competence that we spoke about, attributes associated with character and agency also impact other relationships between healthcare stakeholders.

> Diya is a mid -level executive of a population health company that supports Health Insurance Plans. We asked Diya to give an example of an interaction that created trust in her mind. Diya immediately shared the following story: "I had the opportunity to "pitch" our company and solution to a CEO and the Chief Medical Officer of prominent Health Plan. I was initially a bit intimidated due to their stature. Very quickly the sales presentation became a lively conversation. At the end of the hour, the CEO walked up to me and stated that not only did he find the conversation enjoyable, but he was also very impressed with the solution that we were discussing. He then asked me to send the contract directly to him. I guess that I had a bit of a surprised look on my face. He began to laugh and ask me why I was reacting in such a manner. Without letting me respond he stated, both he personally and his organization likes to work with people that they like, respect and trust. He stated that our conversation made it clear that he could trust both me and the organization that I was representing." She finished the story by telling us that this contractual relationship is now in its fifth year.

Clearly both competence and character are important cornerstones of the trust equation. The question that many ask is "How do I get the information about one's professional and interpersonal skills?" Historically, we received some of this information from friends, family, neighbors, and colleagues. These were the people we trusted for referrals. Unfortunately, societal events such as those that we identified earlier have impacted our trust in our communities and work peers. If we do not trust those people now, what is next? In fact, in our survey we are seeing changes. We asked our respondents, "since the 2016 election do you trust your friends and neighbors more, less or the same." Although most of the sample showed no change 14% said less and only 8 % more. We think this difference is worthy of concern.

Although distinctly different, when it comes to trust, competence and conscience are integrated and intertwined in the equation. If a patient is looking for a doctor to act in our best interest, it this due to competence or consciousness? This is where there is not a clear differentiati on.

# Physician Relationship: Competence and Caring

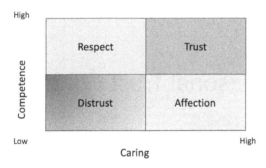

Source: Paling J. Strategies to help patients understand risks. British Medical Journal 2003, 327; pp745-748

The second method of trust typing that we will look at focuses on the participants associated within the trust equation. The most common model utilized with this focus include:

1. Personal Trust
2. Interpersonal Trust
3. Society, System or Organizational Trust

The term personal trust points to the ability of an individual to trust oneself. Am I capable or able to participate in the action being asked of me? Do I believe in myself? One's ability to trust in oneself allows you to both build your own confidence as well as allows you to trust others and others to trust you. In regard to self-trust, we heard two viewpoints from consumers in regard to their own care. The first were those that felt a lack of trust in themselves and their competence to care for themselves.

Josiah was a good example of response. Josiah has type 2 diabetes. Josiah's provider gave him a list of 7 things that he needed to do in order to care for his diabetes. His provider went over the list and instructions and told him to come back in 6 months. Josiah left his providers office overwhelmed, frustrated and angry. "My doctor has studied years to be a doctor and to know what to do for type 2 diabetes. What makes him think that I am prepared to do this on my own? No way!"

## Personal Trust Continuum

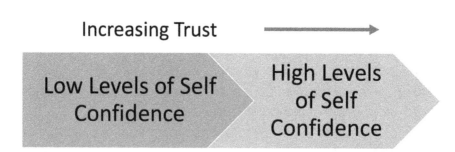

Source: Health Intelligence Partners

The second common response could be considered on the other side of the self confidence and trust continuum. Several people that we spoke to take the viewpoint that "if my doctor is asking me to take on more responsibility then this condition and its requirements must not be that hard."

> Jessie, a 28-year-old woman with newly diagnosed asthma, shared her reaction to her provider discussing how she should take her medications, change her home environment, and monitor her condition. Jessie stated that she trusted her doctor when he said that she could effectively and safely make changes to her medication depending on the circumstances. She also shared that initially she consulted the internet when she had questions. She also shared that she regularly used YouTube to make home repairs. "I am a college graduate; I know how to read, and I know how to take care of myself."

Personal trust is not just an issue for the health consumer, it is also a very real topic for health providers. When a doctor is sued what happens? Does the doctor lose trust in herself as competent?

> Josephine shared that she had been practicing medicine for approximately 10 years. Unfortunately, Josephine was sued by a patient. This patient was someone that she had seen for many years and thought that she had a good relationship with. The experience of being named in a malpractice suit created a situation where she lost trust in herself and considered quitting medicine. It took Josephine a number of years to regain the trust in her ability to practice good medicine even though the malpractice suit was eventually dropped.

Interestingly, personal or self -trust does not just impact how we feel about ourselves and our self-efficacy and confidence, it also can impact whether others trust us and whether we trust others. This is often one of the parameters of interpersonal trust. Science has shown that those that do not have trust in themselves often have difficulty trusting others (Lewicki et al). In the case of Josephine, the question becomes

27

whether her lack of self -trust impacted how her patients felt about her. Does the patient then lose trust for her as a doctor?

The second interaction involving trust in this trust typography is interpersonal trust. Interpersonal trust is the trust between two individuals. This is the type of trust we most commonly refer to in healthcare. This can be between the consumer and their provider, between two providers, a provider, and a healthcare executive or two healthcare executives. In order for trust to occur between two people, one needs to overcome potential vulnerability, informational asymmetry, assumed but unknown intention, and dependence. (Rowe R, Calnan M, Trust Relations in Healthcare- the New Agenda, European Journal of Public health, 16(1)2006. Overcoming these barriers requires one to believe that the competence and character of the other individual can be trusted.

The third interaction in this trust typology model is that of societal, system or organizational trust. Human biology often makes this trust the most difficult. As we discussed earlier, humans are wired to trust another person. This is not necessarily the case with inanimate objects or organizations.

> Jorie, a 33-year-old was asked to name an organization that she trusted. Her answer was intriguing. She stated, "I do not trust any organization. Organizations have no heart and no soul. The reality is that I may trust someone that works in an organization but in most cases that trust does not extend to the organization as a whole."

Jorie's comments align with those that we see in the International survey shown below (Axios). That said, there were a few people that did share their trust in an organization. In many cases this trust was either based on reputation or a personal experience.

Stephano is a 59-year-old that asked what company he trusts the most; he immediately answered that none come to mind at this time, but in the past, he trusted Volvo, the car maker. When asked why he stated that "for many years it was the only make of car that I would allow my children to ride in." As we delved further into this belief, he shared that this trust was associated with two factors; the reputation of the car and the fact that he had been involved in a car accident earlier in his life while driving a Volvo. Neither he nor his passenger were injured.

## Share of people that trust their country's institutions

Online survey of 1,200 adults in select countries. January 2020 survey conducted Oct. 19 to Nov. 18, 2019. May 2020 conducted April 15-23, 2020.

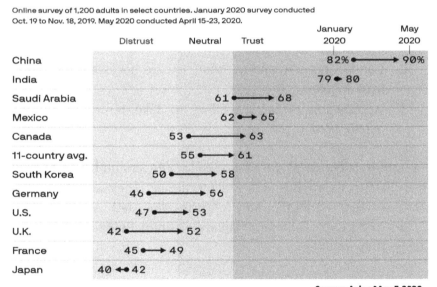

|  | Distrust | Neutral | Trust | January 2020 | May 2020 |
|---|---|---|---|---|---|
| China |  |  |  | 82% ⟶ | 90% |
| India |  |  |  | 79 ⟵ 80 |  |
| Saudi Arabia |  | 61 ⟶ 68 |  |  |  |
| Mexico |  | 62 ⟶ 65 |  |  |  |
| Canada | 53 ⟶ 63 |  |  |  |  |
| 11-country avg. | 55 ⟶ 61 |  |  |  |  |
| South Korea | 50 ⟶ 58 |  |  |  |  |
| Germany | 46 ⟶ 56 |  |  |  |  |
| U.S. | 47 ⟶ 53 |  |  |  |  |
| U.K. | 42 ⟶ 52 |  |  |  |  |
| France | 45 ⟶ 49 |  |  |  |  |
| Japan | 40 ⟷ 42 |  |  |  |  |

**Source: Axios May 5, 2020**

As you can see, about half of the individuals surveyed in the U.S. either distrusted or were neutral regarding organizations and institutions within the country.

Earlier, we discussed the fact that historically healthcare was based on the relationship between the doctor and consumer. Over the last forty years, the healthcare milieu has expanded beyond the provider and the consumer to a number of different organizations including hospitals, health Insurance organizations and organizations that offer health services. As we will discuss later in the book, consumers react to healthcare organizations in a similar manner as to how they react to non-healthcare organizations.

A third commonly utilized trust typography was articulated by Cokie and Steven Roberts. When asked about their definition of trust, they broke it down into 3 elements. (Trust, Shore Harvard)

1. Service- this is not just a simple action but one that has impact and meaning to an individual or group. Value has become a recent touchstone concept in healthcare but one that carries a great deal of weight.
2. Candor- honesty and transparency are necessary for one to trust another.
3. Accountability- being willing to take responsibility and accountability.

A fourth trust typology was identified by Zenger and his co-authors in a 2019 Harvard Business Review article. They also utilized a three -element model that they felt was associated with trust. (Jack Zenger and Joseph Folkman, Harvard Business Review, February 5, 2019). They include:

1. Positive relationships- individuals showing concern for others, cooperation, and honesty
2. Judgement and expertise-knowledgeable
3. Consistency between what you say you will do and what you do.

The fifth and final trust typology that we would like to present consists of:

- Expectant or presumptive trust. This is when we enter an interaction for the first time but through past experiences in a similar situation, trust occurs. Expectant trust in healthcare can be associated with past experience in healthcare or trust in the world in general.
- Experiential trust is associated with trust that occurs over time
- Identification trust is based on two people have shared values and goals.

This trust typology utilizes a unique model that focuses on trust associated with one's experiences either personally or societally. It recognizes that trust builds upon itself.

> Silvia, a 51-year-old woman shared that "of course I trust all of my doctors and nurses. They have always treated me and my family with respect. They take care of our illnesses so that we can continue to live our lives."

Silvia's experience can be seen as either presumptive trust or experiential trust depending on whether she is speaking about providers that she and her family have seen in the past versus her trust in a provider that she has not seen before.

Identification trust has taken on greater importance over the last several years due to increasing research done in the field of demographic and cultural trust and distrust. We will go into greater depth as in the next two sections of the book when we meet Josephine, Amad, Aki and Santiago, as well as discuss two significant events that have created a trust reset, the 2016 election and the 2020 COVID 19 pandemic.

## Measuring Trust and What the Numbers Say

As we have set the foundation of trust through both definition and importance, it is now time to spend a few minutes discussing how to measure trust. Should organizations measure trust? Helen Leis, a Partner in Health and Life Sciences at Oliver Wyman spoke about the importance of measuring trust in healthcare. She is not alone in believing in the importance of measuring trust. Several different measurements have been used over the last 50 years. Leis goes on to articulate the confusion that often occurs between quality measures and experience measures associated with trust. "Both areas impact trust in the healthcare system and those that are in it, but you have to remember that they are different." Leis' comments are important because one needs to be clear as to what they are measuring in order to make sense of the results and then to act on those results in an effective manner. It is also important to differentiate measures focused on satisfaction versus trust. The two are not the same, they are connected, but trust is a proactive feeling and satisfaction is a retrospective feeling looking backward at past action or activity. Satisfaction has also been found to have less of a charged connotation and component than trust, which is more strongly tied to an emotional response. (Thom et al, 2004)

Like almost everything associated with trust, there is no clear agreement on how to measure trust and what to measure. Trust is difficult to quantify, and no specific formulas and calculations exist. That being said, there are a number of organizations that have measured trust either directly or indirectly. The methods of measuring trust vary widely due to the many definitions and varied frameworks associated with the concept. Some correlate well to outcomes and others have not focused on that type of correlation (Thom et al, 2004). There have been some measures that utilize only one question, other short form questionnaires that utilize 5 measures such as the Wake Forest Trust Scale.

A systematic review of surveys focused on trust within the healthcare environment found 45 measurement methodologies associated with trust, again the length varied. A large number of the measurement instruments focused on providers and patients although some focused on other areas of healthcare such as Health Insurance, hospitals or medical research. Very few focused on the system as a whole. (Ozawa)

The lack of agreement should not deter us from measuring trust. As you can see from this last section, trust carries great importance in healthcare. You have probably heard the term "that what is measured, matters." We believe that the flipside is also true. That which matters, needs to be measured. By measuring trust, we highlight its importance. In addition to showing its importance, measurement also allows us to monitor and change management in order to move in the direction of increasing trust within healthcare.

Healthcare has measured trust for over 50 years. Russell Caterinicchio is an early pioneer of measuring trust in healthcare. In 1979 he wrote a paper that focused on the patient-physician trust equation. This paper was considered pivotal because up until that time, it was assumed that patients always trusted their doctors. This was a wakeup call to an industry and the beginning of the breakdown of the trust assumption. This study began a 50-year pattern of various measurement modalities on patient trust specifically and trust within healthcare more broadly. (Thom et al, 2004). Some of these surveys are done in a point of time while others have been done on a regular basis. Organizations such as Pew, Gallup, Edelman and Revive have been measuring trust within healthcare for a number of years. These longitudinal surveys can be helpful to see how relationships and trust have changed over the years. None of these surveys are exactly alike. That being said, patterns exist and there is information that can be acted on in order to positively impact trust. We are going to spend a few minutes looking the data from a few of these organizations and then share with you the results of our measurement survey.

## Edelman

Edelman is an organization that has built a reputation for their focus on trust. Edelman is a global communications company that works to support organizations brands and reputations. As part of their work, Edelman has done an annual trust and credibility survey across institutions, sectors, and geographies since 2012. Edelman uses four dimensions of trust in order to create its Net Trust Score. These four dimensions include Ability, which in this book we call competence, integrity, dependability, and purpose. The Edelman trust barometer reaches out to 500 individuals over the age of 18 in a number of countries including the United States and China. The Edelman Trust Barometer asks the consumer to focus the trust issues on industries as a whole. A few key facts over the last few years include:

- The 2017 Trust Barometer found that:
  » The United States is a nation divided with little trust found across industries.
  » Trust within healthcare, unlike some other surveys done, found that younger adults were more trusting in healthcare as a whole.
  » Decline in trust in business, government, and media. A bit better news for healthcare.
  » The reduction in trust is moderating. That being said, trust measures are poor as well and decreasing. Some would say "can't fall off the floor." The only industry that is worse than healthcare is the government. The study found that healthcare as an industry puts profit above people.
- The 2018 Trust Barometer found that in the year between the 2017 and 2018 survey there was:
  » a 10% decrease in the trust of all businesses. A large percentage of those surveyed stated that "CEOs are driven by greed more than making a positive difference"
  » 14% decrease in the trust of government

- » 5% decrease in the trust of all forms of media
- » 3% decrease in the trust of "persons like yourself." Overall friends and peers are losing credibility and trust and that they had a" lack of confidence in trust"
- The 2019 Trust Barometer
  - » Significant widening gap in trust between healthcare stakeholders although there was a 4% overall increase in trust in the industry as a whole
  - » Women trust less than men and this continues to expand. It is believed that women trust less than men at a 15 % gap due to the fact that women overall trust business less than men. This is due to a variety of issues including pay inequality and the recent #MeToo, movement, issues associated with the "glass ceiling," and how women often feel as if they are treated as second tier citizens. This lack of trust by women is important as women most often act as the lead of the family's healthcare decisions. (CEO of the household and healthcare)
  - » There is an increasing gap in trust between those that are considered informed and the mass population by a 10% gap
  - » Hospitals and clinics saw a 1% reduction in trust between 2018 and 2019, whereas biotech saw a 1% increase, health insurance saw a 2% increase and pharmaceutical companies saw a 4% increase in trust. It is important to remember that these three areas have had low trust scores over the last few years and have struggled with trust, especially pharma.

## Oliver Wyman

Oliver Wyman, a strategic consultancy that offers advice in both healthcare and life sciences conducted a Consumer Health Survey of 2,016 Americans regarding their experiences with the healthcare system. The Oliver Wyman questionnaire asks a series of questions that are more specific to the healthcare industry than the Edelman Trust Index. The following were findings from their study:

- All generations of individuals surveyed found healthcare complex and confusing.
- All found the rising costs of healthcare a concern. When comparing retailers to healthcare, 34% of consumers were willing to recommend a general retailer; 24% a tech company; 20% a retail pharmacy; 2% a health insurance company and -8% a hospital.
- In regard to the cost of healthcare, 43% want their doctor to make a healthcare decision on their behalf as if the cost was their own, 28% wanted whatever was best for their health, regardless of cost; 21% wanted the information about how much their care was going to cost but would make the decision on their own; and 8% wanted to doctor to recommend the least expensive care possible.
- Overall, consumers were willing to share their health data. Only 11% that would not be willing to share under any circumstances

## Gallup

Gallup, an organization that is known to many consumers, utilizes analytics in order to help identify areas of focus across organizations, both public and private. Gallup has surveyed the public over a number of years regarding American's viewpoint on healthcare. Most of the Gallup surveys include approximately 1000 Adult age Americans

The 2015 Gallup Survey on Health and Healthcare interviewed individuals about their healthcare found that:

- only 37% of those asked had confidence in the medical system.

- In general, 65% were satisfied with their healthcare. Although this number remained over 50%, the trend was downward from the previous year's survey (67%).
- Most people trusted their healthcare providers to be honest and ethical; with nurses being rated the highest at 84%, pharmacists at 67% and doctors at 65%. Interestingly nurses have rated highest for honesty for every year but once since 1999
    » Nurses 85%
    » Physicians 65%
    » Pharmacists 64%
    » Dentists 61%
    » Chiropractors 41%
    » Journalists 28%
    » Business executives 20%
    » Members of Congress 12%

The 2017 Survey on Health and Healthcare found that:

- Healthcare was their "greatest worry," with a focus on both access and affordability
- People get healthcare information from the internet 43% of the time. (Gallup)
- People trust their physicians more than their spouses, family and friends in regard to health although family is a greater motivator than their doctor. Other places that can impact an individual and their health through trust include
    » Primary care physician 43%
    » Place of worship 29%
    » People in general 27%
    » Health plan 22%
    » Employer 13%
    » Personal health coach 12%

The 2018 Gallup Poll on Health and Healthcare:

- 70% of individuals surveyed stated that the American health-care system was "in a state of crisis" or having "major problems" (McCarthy, J. Seven in 10 Maintain Negative View of U.S. Healthcare System. Wellbeing. January 14, 2018)

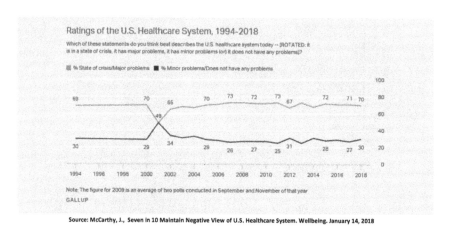

Source: McCarthy, J., Seven in 10 Maintain Negative View of U.S. Healthcare System. Wellbeing. January 14, 2018

# Revive

Revive Healthcare, a service company that focuses their work on the intersection of healthcare delivery, finance and innovation in order to support clients and the healthcare industry, has been doing the Revive Health Trust Index since 2006. For 10 years the Trust Index was focused on business-to-business trust within the healthcare industry. The Revive Health Trust Index is a 100 -point survey that utilizes fairness, reliability and honesty into a composite score. In 2017 the Trust Index expanded to include the healthcare consumer. The 2017 Index found that there was a lack of trust across all stakeholders within healthcare. A few specific findings include:

- Health plans have more trust in providers (hospitals and doctors) at 67% than providers have in health plans 54%.

- 79% of patients stated that they trusted their doctors and that that doctors were mostly honest
- 74% of patients stated that they trust their hospitals
- 69% of patients stated that they trust their insurance companies. They stated that they felt "slighted by their health plans"

## The Physicians' Foundation

The Physicians' Foundation is a nonprofit organization that seeks to strengthen the physician and patient relationship. Unlike the surveys listed above the Physicians Foundation Survey focuses entirely on the provider and the consumer by identifying how physicians and patients feel about the healthcare system. The survey is done on a biennial basis. The 2018 Survey focused on the patient and physician relationship. Although 95% of the patients surveyed were satisfied with their primary care provider

- 90% said that true partnership is the most essential element of quality
- 11% said that they had adequate time with their provider
- 90% stated that physicians must take the lead on behalf of their patients when it comes to cost and quality issues. In contrast, 69% of those surveyed felt that the insurance companies today have the greatest influence in these issues.
- 89% of patients are afraid that the cost of their care will adversely impact them in the future. To that end, 19% have skipped doses of medications due to cost and 25% did not fill at least one medication due to cost
- 82% of the patients surveyed believe that physicians should provide access to their electronic medical records
- 57% feel that their physician relies more on what the computer tells them then what the patient is saying
- 77% wish that their doctor would listen to them more

## Pew

The Pew Research Foundation is a nonpartisan think tank that regularly does public opinion polling and other forms of research in order to inform the public on issues that shape who we are and what we do as a country. A number of Pew surveys have looked at both trust as a factor of action and reaction in areas of healthcare that affect a consumer's trust.

A Pew Research Center Survey from August 2, 2017 found that:

- 26% of those surveyed felt that the U.S. healthcare system is above average compared to other healthcare systems in the world
- 23% of patients that saw their physician in the last year felt rushed and not listened to
- 80% of patients that saw their physician in the last year felt that they did get the information that they needed about the treatment that they were receiving
- 15% felt very confused about the instructions that they were given

A more recent Pew Research Survey of 2019 found that:

- 75% of Americans trust in the federal government and this number has been decreasing.
- 64% of Individuals stated that they trust others. This too has been decreasing.
- Those surveyed stated that their low level of trust makes it harder to solve problems in federal government and solving problems harder with those that they deal with on a regular basis.
- Most of those surveyed don't trust many of the individuals that have positions of power in the U.S. due to their low rates of empathy, transparency and ethics.
- 64% of those surveyed believe that peoples' trust in each other has been declining due to increasing greed and dishonesty and

that this makes it harder to solve problems. When breaking down these figures to demographics it was found that non -whites, less educated and younger adults skew towards greater distrust.

## The Harris Poll

The Harris Poll is an organization that utilizes information from survey to reveal the values and concerns of modern society. In 2016 Harris did a survey with 1000 adults over the age of 18 that identified those healthcare organizations with low and high reputations. What they found aligned with other organizations

# Organizational Reputation

| Industry | Percent Low reputation | Percent High reputation |
|---|---|---|
| Health Insurance | 24 | 15 |
| Pharmaceutical Manufacturer | 20 | 20 |
| Hospitals | 6 | 37 |
| Doctors/Providers | 5 | 43 |

Source: Harris Poll, 2016

The survey also showed that patients do not see anyone protecting their interest which leads to lack of consumer trust:

- 9% of consumers believe that pharmaceutical manufacturers and biotech organizations put patients over profits
- 10% of consumers believe Health Insurance Companies put patients over profits
- 36% of consumers believe that doctors put patients over profits

## The Health Intelligence Partners Healthcare Trust Survey

Health Intelligence Partners is a Healthcare Consultancy focused on the intersection of clinical, analytical and operational strategy. In 2017 we performed our first trust survey, using electronic distribution, and received results on 1,161 participants randomly distributed over the United States. The survey focused on a wide range of questions around trust in healthcare. Specifically, patient focused questions on trust in their doctor, trust in other health care providers, trust in the healthcare system and trust in the data collected in health care. (see charts below)

The survey showed that:

- Overwhelming trust in a patient's own physician for sharing information at 92%, with no close second (person or entity)
- Overwhelming trust in a patient's own physician at 89% for treatment advice, with no close second (person or entity)
- When asked why a patient trusted their doctor, it came down to two main reasons:
  » "how they treat me" 74%
  » "how they talk to me"77%
- When asked if their level of trust in the healthcare system had changed since the election in 2016
  » 35% said they trusted the healthcare system less
  » 4% of respondents trusted their own physician less.
  » 18% stated that they trusted their friends and neighbors less

As you can see, each of these organizations place a different emphasis within their trust surveys depending on their focus. Although, the specific results vary, the general output and trends do not. We have a trust problem. Trust across healthcare is low with even worsening trends. One of the most interesting insights to arise during the interview portion of our work was their surprise about the results of our research regarding the lack of trust that existed regarding across all of the stakeholder groups in healthcare.

We believe the next steps to re-engaging in trust is to take the data from the surveys presented above as well as others that were not mentioned, identify some of the major stakeholders within the health-care environment and address specific actions, or trust resets ™, that should be considered. Without this specific focus on improving trust within and across healthcare, regardless of all of the changes that we are making in creating new organizational structures and alternative financing models, we will not achieve the goals of improved access, quality and cost that we are looking the attain

## % Trust my physician/doctor

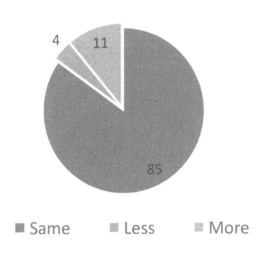

Same    Less    More

Source: Health Intelligence Partners Trust Survey, 2018
N=1161

# % Trust Health Care System

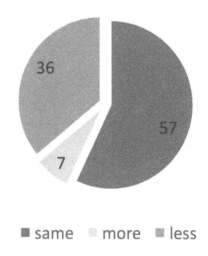

■ same   ■ more   ■ less

**Source: Health Intelligence Partners Trust Survey, 2018**
**N=1161**

# % Trust friends and neighbors

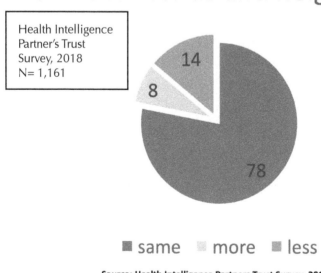

Health Intelligence
Partner's Trust
Survey, 2018
N= 1,161

■ same   ■ more   ■ less

**Source: Health Intelligence Partners Trust Survey, 2018**
**N=1161**

# For those who said they did not trust their doctor...

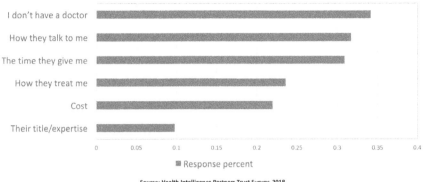

Source: Health Intelligence Partners Trust Survey, 2018
N=1161

Over 34% of respondents who did not trust their doctor did so because they reported they did not have a physician. However, for the rest "how they talked to me" and "the time they gave me" were the top responses (32%, 31%). These responses are very interesting and seem to focus on some critical issues that we understand in healthcare. First, physicians are under pressure to bill for treatment. Thus, spending time with their patient takes a backseat to collecting data for their EHR and getting more patients in the door. Second, very little time is spent educating physicians to maximize their emotional quotient (EQ). Due to this, negative interactions feel rushed. We might also suggest that "how they talk with me" would be based on the rushed interactions and potentially a more technical/less personal approach to care.

# Section Two:
# The Stakeholders

"When you talk about trust you must know the way a group thinks, interacts, communicates, and educates. You have to understand their roles and relationships. What are their values? Their practices? What are the expected behaviors?"

Phyllis Pettit Nassi

Trust is the lubrication necessary for a successful interaction no matter who the individuals are or what role they play. Healthcare is no different. Trust is central to all relationships. Earlier we spoke about how the Merriam- Webster Medical Dictionary talks about trust being "a concept involving both confidence and reliance." This is true in healthcare as it is in society.

Broad societal or social trust is the underpinning of the more specific trust that occurs within healthcare. Pew social trends defines societal trust as the "belief in the honesty, integrity and reliability of others, this is often known as "faith in people." (Pew Research Center; Americans and Social Trust: Who, Where and Why. Feb. 2007)

A February 2019 Aspen Institute Program focusing on Media and Democracy stated that the nation is in a "crisis of trust." They are not alone in this belief. The Pew survey found that a large number (50%) of individuals felt that you cannot be too careful and 30% believed that others would try and take advantage of them. Our data found that 20% of individuals did not trust their friends, family or neighbors.

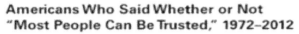

**Americans Who Said Whether or Not
"Most People Can Be Trusted," 1972–2012**

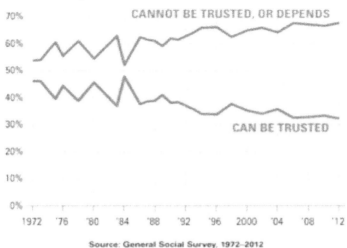

Source: General Social Survey, 1972–2012

The factors that have brought us to this point are not new. Trust challenges have existed for many years. The book "Consequences of Modernity" goes into depth explaining that as societies mature, trust decreases. Although there have been times with reduced friction and less obvious trust challenges, the situation continues to exist and has been increasing over the last 60 years. A great deal of this began in the 1960's with the Viet Nam war. In addition to the Viet Nam war, the decade was challenged by counter cultural events that produced one of the most memorable sayings from the 1960s "don't trust anyone over thirty" coined by Jack Weinberg. Although this trust challenge was focused on age, the distrust from those years have continued to mount. Factors such as socioeconomics differences, geographic locations, cultural, race and religions have played a role in creating trust challenges. Politics is one factor that adds significant "fuel to the fire" of distrust. Since the late 1970s the United States population has become more polarized across political ideologies and parties. This issue is not confined to one political party or another. A 2019 Pew study that showed that this decrease in trust in government has had broad implications to overall trust in the United States, impacting how much people trust each other in general. Forty-nine percent of those that were surveyed stated that this decrease in personal trust can be attributed to people not being as reliable as they use to be. One individual surveyed by Pew stated that "we have lost confidence in each other." This overall societal decrease in trust has created an atmosphere of distrust across most institutions.

This trust challenge has spread to healthcare. One would hope that personal differences, whether they are based on political and ideologic beliefs, physical features, racial or cultural differences would not affect our health and healthcare. The Hippocratic Oath speaks to its impartiality by stating, "into whatsoever house I enter, I will help the sick". The Declaration of Geneva created in 1946 by the World Medical Association, updated in 2017, once again stated the impartiality of care by stating, "I will not permit considerations of age, disease, disability, creed, ethnic origin, gender, nationality, political affiliation, race, sexual orientation, social standing or other factor to intervene between my duty and my patient". (Berwick D. Polititcs and Healthcare, JAMA, October 9, 2018)

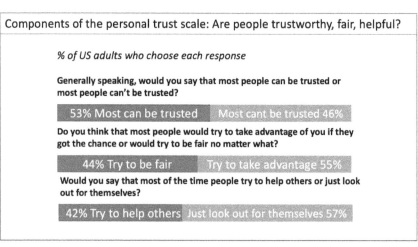

Components of the personal trust scale: Are people trustworthy, fair, helpful?

*% of US adults who choose each response*

Generally speaking, would you say that most people can be trusted or most people can't be trusted?

53% Most can be trusted    Most cant be trusted 46%

Do you think that most people would try to take advantage of you if they got the chance or would try to be fair no matter what?

44% Try to be fair    Try to take advantage 55%

Would you say that most of the time people try to help others or just look out for themselves?

42% Try to help others  Just look out for themselves 57%

Source: Pew Research, March 2020

We need to ask ourselves who bears responsibility within the health-care environment to take the lead and address the trust challenge? Realistically, trust is a shared responsibility. Each of us plays a role in the trust equation. Historically, this was a much simpler problem to solve as the stakeholders consisted of the patient (in some cases also their families, especially in pediatrics), the doctor and their staff. Today, the health and healthcare industry have a large and diverse stakeholder environment. In addition, the stakeholders, both traditional and non-traditional, are growing exponentially.

In Section 1, we discussed the existence of different types of trust. You will note, as we discuss the different stakeholders that participate in the health and healthcare environment that many of these types of trust will come into play. The dynamics associated with human interaction have an impact on whether trusting interactions and relationships exist. These interactions include but are not limited to cooperation, competition, personalities and communication styles, past experience, institutional hierarchies, and individual backgrounds. We must remember that the healthcare system is made of individuals. When individuals don't believe that the system is working with and for them, they do not trust that system. At initial read, you may believe that this is the case specifically between the patient and the healthcare system. The reality is this feeling extends far beyond that of the healthcare consumer into individuals across the continuum. You will hear this rhetoric from patients, providers, and executives. All individuals carry with them attributes that influence how they interact and how they trust. Let's take a few minutes to focus on some of these attributes.

## The Stakeholder as an Individual: Demographics Have an Impact on Trust

Trust is biologically wired into all of us but that does not mean that we are alike in how much we trust, who we trust and the impact on trust. Each of us is made up of a number of characteristics. These characteristics include our general demographics, our education, our socio-economic status, our country of origin and where we reside now, and our race, and past experience to name just a few. Each of these features affect how we feel, think and act. They also influence how we interact and who we trust. It is important that we recognize how demographics can play a role in trust.

## Age

"Never trust anyone over 30"
Jack Weinberg 1964

The impact of age on trust is a social phenomenon that is not new. This statement came about as Jack was speaking to the San Francisco Chronicle. His words reflected the youth movement's lack of trust for "the establishment" and authority. Over time the meaning expanded to include not only organizational and societal ageism but also a lack of trust of individuals over the age of 30. Jack Weinberg's 1964 historic statement, as well as the social and societal movement of the 1960s, encouraged distrust across age lines. Here we are in 2020 and the question of age and trust remains. Unfortunately, the answer to the question of age correlation to trust is not clear due to conflicting data. Pew Research Center found that younger Americans (ages 18-29) have low levels of trust in general. This information correlates with a number of other studies that found younger people were overall less trusting of their providers, hospitals, the government, and the healthcare system as a whole. Research done by Michael Polin in 2015 found that after taking into account a number of other individual factors, age does make a "notable difference in trust." The study went on to state that when asked if "most people can be trusted" 23% of 20-year-olds agreed whereas 35% of those over the age of 80 agreed. (Poulin, 2015)). Another study, this one by the Pew Foundation showed young adults had had a lack of trust in institutions in general and the healthcare system in specific. Like the Pew and Poulin study, our study found that those individuals under the age of 45 had a lower level of trust in their providers than those over the age if 45 years old. Our qualitative studies were able to give us a greater understanding of some of the issues that we believe impact one's trust in healthcare and their age. There are three themes that seem to be most prominent to those under the age of 45. These include:

1. Lack of trust in institutions as a whole. In this case, healthcare is bundled into larger societal and institutional distrust.
2. Belief that healthcare should be a right and should be covered by the government as a single payer model.
3. Health as a broader definition and theme. It is more common for younger individuals to think of health more broadly. This demographic tends to use alternative providers and activities to address their health and healthcare needs.

The Health Intelligence Partners data showed that trust in one's primary care physician grew with age. The group with the highest level of trust was those that were 60+ (94%). This data is similar to many other studies. It is likely that this high level of trust for this demographic group is associated with the historical belief that an individual should "listen" to their doctor. We found that those that we spoke to over the age of 50 were often brought up to believe the following

1. Respect for the healthcare field
2. Trust based on competency of doctors and other healthcare professionals
3. Presumed good intent of those in the healthcare field

## GENDER

There have been numerous studies regarding the impact of gender on issues of trust. The results of these studies often conflict with each other. There are a number of reasons for conflicting results including:

a. The questions that were asked in the study
b. The time period in which the study was done
c. Areas of trust that were studied

Although we will not go into depth on these studies, we want to take a moment to address the issue of timing. As we discussed earlier in the book, societal events often have a significant impact on trust. Over the last four years there has been increasing degradation of trust in societal institutions. The 2019 Edelman Trust Barometer research quantified how this general societal trend specifically impacted women's level of trust. The study found that women are less trusting of institutions and business than men. The reasons for this attitude include their continued frustration with the lack of necessary change in both society as a whole and more specifically in business. This phenomenon is not specific to the United States. Women's frustration and lack of trust is international, however, these sentiments are more common in the U.S. The "me- too" movement has only increased women's mistrust. Organizations that take the need for change seriously and act upon that need are regaining the trust of women. Unfortunately, unlike business, healthcare has failed to demonstrate the desire to make many of these changes. Therefore, women continue to show high levels of distrust in the healthcare system.

In addition to societal issues, there are other reasons for gender differences in regard to trust. In the book, Men are From Mars, Women are From Venus, John Gray talks about psychological differences between men and women. (Gray, 1992). He states that these differences can have significant impact on the relationships they form and subsequent trust between the sexes. Some of these differences are tied to communication styles while others are associated with belief styles. Research has also shown that the communication differences between men and women can affect the type of relationships built, and the formation of trust within these relationships. (Furumo,2007)

When speaking of the impact of gender on trust, it is important to differentiate between trusting another individual versus being trustworthy as an individual. Further studies have shown that gender's impact on trust is inconsistent. A number of studies have shown that men trust more than women, but women are more trustworthy than men.

There are some that believe that this lack of trust by women is similar to other demographic groups that have historically been discriminated against. (Buchan, 2008). Overall, those that have the historical experience of discrimination are less likely to believe that others can be trusted. (Buchan, 2008)

Our study contradicted a number of the other studies that have been done as we found that women have more confidence in the healthcare system than males. In addition, women trust their providers more than men do (90% v 88%). What we heard during our interviews gave us a bit of insight into why women showed a greater level of trust.

> Lilly, a 45-year-old woman stated that she was responsible for her entire family's healthcare needs, including her parents, her husband's parents, her husband and her 3 children. "If I did not trust people to take care of us, my role as the healthcare decision maker would be too hard. I am not sure if I really trust the system and the doctors or if I am just making assumptions so that I can oversee all of this.

## Younger Generation is "dissatisfied" or "very dissatisfied" with aspects of traditional health care

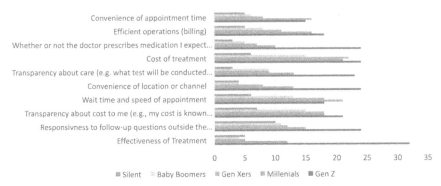

Source: Adapted from, "http://www.Accenture.com/us-en/insights/health/todays-consumers-reveal-future-healthcare

## Socio-economic Status (SES)

Jeremy, a 51 year-old who has worked in restaurants most of his life shared with us his thoughts on how socio-economic status impacts trust. Jeremy started out by stating that he had finally found a provider that treated him in a similar fashion to how he treated other people. When I asked Jeremy to explain what he meant he shared that he felt that other providers that he had seen looked down at him. "I finished college; you know. I just never found a job that I really liked. I love food and figured I might as well spend my time around something that I am passionate about. Unfortunately, it has left me living from paycheck to paycheck. When I go to see a doctor, they assume I am stupid. They figure that I don't understand what they are saying. It hard to trust someone that looks down at you. When I found this new doctor, he treated me like an equal. He explained things and asked for my opinion. I believe in this doctor."

It is disappointing to think that one's socio-economic status should have an impact on the trust between a healthcare consumer and their providers. Unfortunately, many of the studies have shown that this is the case. Nicholas Arpey and his colleagues found that socio-economic status does impact how two people inter-relate. The study found that most consumers believe that their socioeconomic status affected the healthcare that they received. Issues such as access to care, treatment options available to them and their past healthcare interactions have all been articulated reasons that they don't trust their doctors or the healthcare system to offer them high quality care. One example documented in the paper was how people of lesser SES believed that they were prescribed generic medications while those of higher SES received brand name drugs. Although most studies have found SES to have an impact on trust of the healthcare system, there are a few studies that have found that SES has little or no impact on trust. Guerrero and her co-authors found that SES was not associated with trust in healthcare. The authors contend that the reason for this is that those with a similar SES status differ in other ways and that those other attributes play a greater role. (Guerrero, 2015)

Socio-economic status as a factor in how two individuals react is not just found in the consumer/provider relationship, it is also found to be a co-founding factor between providers as well as between healthcare executives. It is unclear whether the issue is socio- economic status alone or other professional factors such as title.

> Delphine is a Chief Medical Officer of a large national organization. When Delphine bought a new car, the other senior executives looked down at her. They told her that her choice of cars is a way to show that she has gotten to an important level of status. They stated that they could not trust her if she did not understand "the rules of the game"

## CULTURE, RELIGION AND RACE

As we have discussed, trust is most commonly based on communication and relationships. In addition to the factors that we have identified; one's race, religion and culture have been found to carry significant influence on relationships and therefore impact trust. If consumers don't feel safe, don't feel "seen" or respected, it is less likely that they will trust their interactions with others. The reasons for lack of respect vary in each of these three areas.

## Cultural Norms

Our actions and interactions are often driven by cultural norms. Cultural differences can create a trust fracture™ if there is lack of attention and mutual understanding of these social beliefs and practices. Pavneet Singh discussed how cultural discordance negatively impacted the clinical interactions and trust within a South Asian population. A large portion of the population that he studied were found to be non-adherent to the treatment protocols discussed and prescribed by their healthcare providers. The reason for the non-adherence involved a number of cultural issues that were not identified and addressed by their providers such as:

1.  How one greets someone in this culture. The greeting makes a significant impact on the initial rapport and the creation of trust in the healthcare provider. Handshakes, hugs and greetings all impact how the provider is trusted and how the ongoing relationship will proceed.
2.  The "collectivist culture" of South Asians. Whereas many Caucasian cultures are based on an individualistic cultural underpinning, South Asians are more focused on the "us culture." The importance and inclusion of the family plays a significant role in one's healthcare in this population.
3.  The role of traditional medicine and medications for those that are first or second generation South Asian.

## Religion

Strong feelings and affiliations with one's religion can impact their trust in healthcare. In some cases, religion has been found to increase positive feelings towards those individuals that practice within the healthcare due to the respect that healthcare holds in these groups. Studies found that although religion impacted trust at an individual level, it has less impact when measuring trust at an institutional level. (Benjamins 2006)

In other cases, religion may create a barrier of trust because of one's religious beliefs. One such case is when religious doctrine directly conflicts with the treatment that is being recommended. (Curlin, 2005) A second area in which religion and religious beliefs may create a trust fracture™ focuses on the individuals involved.

Mona is a Muslim woman who was seeking gynecological care. She did not have a primary care doctor as she was in her 20s and in good health. She called a Women's health group in the community in which she lived and worked. Mona asked to see a female provider for her care. The individual that took the call for the medical group said that they would be happy to see her, but they could not promise that she would see a woman and that all the providers were competent. Mona explained that it was not about competence but about her cultural and religious beliefs which required her to maintain her modesty by seeing only women providers. The Provider office said that there was nothing that they could do to address her needs. Mona ended up finding another healthcare practitioner after realizing that she could not trust the Women's Health Group due to their lack of sensitivity and respect associated with her religious beliefs around modesty.

## Race and Trust

Race can have a significant impact on the level of trust in the healthcare system. Direct concern about implicit and societal bias has been known to create a barrier to trust. In addition to cultural norms, past experience often impacts how and who trusts in a number of instances including healthcare. An example of this can be found within the Black community where studies have shown consistently that Black consumers trust organizations, including healthcare organizations, less than Caucasians. (Corbie-Smith, Thomas 2002) David Shore, in his book, spoke about the impact of race on trust within healthcare. He found that 15% of Black consumers and 11% of Latinx consumers believe that they would get better care if the were a different race. In 2002, research by Collins found that African Americans did not trust the healthcare system to take care of them as well as they do other individuals of different race. (Collins 2002) One study found that Blacks were 37% less likely to trust their physicians than were Caucasians. (Boulware et al, 2003) The reasons for this lack of trust are complicated.

In the Black community, history has a significant impact on trust of the healthcare community. The historical impact on trust can be due to a person's direct past experience or due to historical issues that did not directly impact the individual. Those that have directly experienced racism are more concerned about trusting the system than those that have not experienced such an event. A Pew Study stated that 71% of Blacks and 63% of Hispanics feel that they were the victim of professional misconduct or racial discrimination from someone in the healthcare system verses 43% of Caucasians (Pew).

There are more nuanced causes of mistrust. As we have discussed, communication is a foundation to building trusting relationships. Monica Peek, in her paper, discusses the issue of Black consumers stating that they experienced poorer communication in regard to their healthcare concerns than Caucasians. This included their physician not listening, not being supportive, not being responsive and not forming the "partnerships" that they felt were necessary to create a trusting relationship. In addition, they felt that Caucasian providers do not understand anything about the experience of being Black. Her research went on to talk specifically about how Black consumers with diabetes have issues around trusting their physicians and others within the healthcare system. This lack of trust impacted their ability to create a safe environment for shared decision making regarding their healthcare in general and their diabetes in specific. (Peek) Baker, in his study found that that it was not only actions that occurred to the individual themself, but also those actions that happened to others in their community or in the past. (Baker et al, 2008)

During our interviews we found that the history of discrimination and lack of honesty across the healthcare system had created a legacy of distrust. Several of the people that we spoke to pointed to the Tuskegee Syphilis Study. The Tuskegee study was funded by the U.S. government and looked to answer the question as to the impact of withholding treatment to individuals diagnosed with syphilis. The subjects enrolled in the study were African American farmers who without consent were injected with syphilis and then had treatment withheld. This unethical experimentation has created an environment where Blacks often believe they are being lied to, deceived or treated" as an experiment." They feel that doctors will not tell the truth and are hiding something.

The demographics and individual aspects discussed here are not the only factors. Other factors such as geographic differences, educational background and health status also tend to form the mosaic of trust . One example of this was articulated in David Shore's book. He found that individuals from the south trust less and have less confidence in the healthcare system than the remainder of the country. (Shore, 2012)

Regardless of differences in religion, culture, race, or other attributes, humans tend to have greater trust in "people like us". Humans are "tribal" by nature. This creates a situationwere we commonly have greater trust in those that share our backgrounds. It is not unusual that there is a racial or cultural discordance between a consumer and their provider. This creates a situation where the consumer often feels that "the provider is not like me" and therefore may have different values than I do or not understand me. One example is the impact of gender concordance between the provider and the healthcare consumer in regard to medication adherence. A 2016 study found that gender discordance decreased trust which created decreased adherence to medication. (Brown, 2016) Gender is not the only type of discordance that has been shown to negatively impact medication adherence due to lack of trust. Country of origin discordance has also been found to have a similar negative impact on medication adherence.

The impact of consumer/provider discordance with gender and country of origin are not the only attributes that have been found to impact trust. The lack of willingness to be vulnerable has been identified in a number of other demographic groups.

George is a 25-year-old gay male that stated that he has very little trust in the healthcare system. Because of this fear and mistrust, will only get his healthcare from Howard Brown Health Clinic in Chicago an LGBTQ focused health center.

If the outcomes of one's care is positive, trust grew. This is another reason why long -term relationships between patients and their physicians have a positive impact on trust.

## The Stakeholders in the Healthcare Trust Equation

"To trust is to allow ourselves to be vulnerable and to be confident in another's intentions."

In addition to the dynamics at an individual level, there are systemic dynamics that come into play. Healthcare is not a solitary sport. In addition to many of the individual attributes listed above, accountability and roles are important in gaining and maintaining trust. As roles change, power changes. Healthcare has been built on a hierarchical system. This can create challenges to trust at an individual level. The reality is that healthcare consists of both individuals, teams, and organizations. Research shows that trust solidifies teams, enables them to run smoothly and reduces possible mistakes. Edelman in their 2017 study stated that "without trust, systems fail." If we do not consciously re-introduce trust, the healthcare system will not produce acceptable results, or it may fail. The power of trust needs to come from many places. It is not single faceted and must be reciprocal in order to make an authentic impact.

Trust, for a variety of reasons, is very important to the patient. Trust is not only important to the patient, but it is also critical for other stakeholders in the healthcare field, but for different reasons.

"Healthcare is like an orchestra. Everyone has to work together in order for the music to work" To sound good, we all have to be aligned and play together. It is a common goal, to make beautiful music." This statement was made by Mark Ganz, the CEO of Cambia Health Solutions.

## The Consumer

Seth, an airline pilot, compared his experience with the whole healthcare system and the individuals he interacted with to the feelings that Bruce McCandless may have felt as the first astronaut to fly untethered in space in 1984. "At times I felt vulnerable and at other times frightened. I just never knew what to expect. In the end, it has always ended up ok, but the not knowing during the journey is really hard."

Over the last several years there has been increased focus on placing the consumer in the center of their own health. This requires the consumer to assume greater personal responsibility and control over their health with the goal of having a positive impact on their clinical and financial health. This is a lofty goal that must be more than just rhetoric. A number of behavior changes need to occur in order for the consumer to transition from a more passive role to an activated role. This transformation will require the consumer to achieve greater levels of self -trust as well as behavior change by the other stakeholders.

As we discussed earlier in the book, self-trust is an important factor in achieving the positive outcomes desired in health and healthcare.

What is trust in one's self? It is commonly recognized as competence or confidence in one's ability to reach a desired goal. Albert Bandura and others have done a great deal of research on how an individual can learn to trust one's self and achieve self-competence (self- efficacy).

The advent of the internet has created one such path towards the democratization of healthcare and self-efficacy. "Dr Google" has become a primary provider of information for many, most commonly in those born after 1982. This path to self- efficacy brings with it, both opportunity and challenges. The good news is that for those that want to be actively engaged, there are methods to do so. The availability of information allows for changes in consumer knowledge, relationships, and power. The downside of easily available information is that it is not always correct. The information on the web can be limited in its scientific foundation, biased in its opinion and in some cases is based on "fake news."

> Dr. Judy is a pediatrician for Steven, a 10-year-old patient that suffered from asthma. Steven's asthma was difficult to control, and Dr. Judy suggested that they begin a course of inhaled steroids. This was discussed with Steven's mother. She asked to have a few days to think about this and discuss this with Steven's father. Steven and his mother returned to see Dr. Judy the next week with 110 pages of information from the internet. Dr Judy was initially thrilled that Steven's mother was so engaged in her son's healthcare. Unfortunately Dr Judy very quickly found that much of the information that Steven's mother had collected and read were from sources with limited scientific evidence. Steven's mother suggested to Dr Judy a number of minerals and other treatments that were not based on good science. She became frustrated that Dr Judy would not follow these alternative treatment models.

This story of Steven's mother and Dr Judy points out a couple of important factors in regard to self- trust. Consumers trust in themselves to be able to communicate their concerns, needs and goals. Knowledge of the science of healthcare is unequal. Individuals study for years to gain knowledge in their field in order to support and direct the patient. Others within the healthcare arena have knowledge and insights in their expertise to guide healthcare through a challenging and changing society. Only the healthcare consumer has the knowledge of what they value and what is important to them when it comes to their health and life.

Another such path is to have someone knowledgeable that we trust helping us to become competent and succeed. Once we are involved in the activity and believe we can be successful, we are more likely to trust ourselves in the future. As Neal Kaufman of Canary Health stated, "mastery experiences lead one to better trust themselves. This is the path to self -efficacy." The phrase "see one, do one, teach one" is often used to articulate how experience and self-trust lead to one's ability to master an act.

Bandura reminds us that in order to gain this self -trust and confidence we need leadership by others that we trust. Trust in that "teacher", whether an individual or an organization, is the only way a patient can show vulnerability, open up to learning, give their information, their bodies, and in fact their life to a healthcare system and those that function within it.

Who is that "teacher" and what allows us to trust them? The 2018 Health Intelligence Survey asked respondents who they trusted to be their "teacher." The survey did not require consumers to choose only one individual, nor did we require respondents to force rank those on the list. The majority of respondents (89%) stated that they trusted doctors to be their lead "teacher" for healthcare advice.

# For healthcare treatment/advice do you trust any of the following (check all that apply)

| Answer | Percent (rounded to nearest 2 digit | N |
|---|---|---|
| My doctor | 89 | 952 |
| My friend | 36 | 275 |
| My pharmacist/pharmacy | 58 | 616 |
| The pharmaceutical manufacturer / maker of medicines that you may take | 9 | 93 |
| My urgent care facility, ED, or retail health clinic (e.g. CVS, Walgreens | 38 | 401 |
| My hospital | 47 | 500 |
| Online, internet or tele-health | 20 | 212 |
| Health insurance provider (e.g. United, BCBS, Aetna) | 13 | 141 |

Source: Health Intelligence Partners Trust Survey, 2018
N=1161

After identifying the trusted teacher or individual we need to discover what allows us as healthcare consumers to trust others. A 2008 New York Times article discusses how consumers have historically had a level of "blind trust" in our doctors (Parker-Pope T, In Doctors We Trust. New York Times December 18, 2008). This issue of "blind trust" is often brought up. We assume competence and character in our healthcare providers. This means that because of the doctor's title and stature the patient trusts the doctor or the person in charge. Regardless, people want a competent doctor that they can trust.

These patients tend to hold providers in very high esteem. This is commonly found in patients that were more likely to prefer a passive role in the relationship. This has been found to be more common in certain cultures and certain ages. (Kraetchmer, Peek) In 1966, 73% of people that were survey stated that they had great confidence in the" leaders of the medical profession" and that they trusted them. It was clear during our interviews that there was a definite population that trusted their providers based on the fact that they were doctors or other licensed professionals.

This also seems to correlate with age. Those individuals that we spoke with that were over 70 were more likely to display blind trust.

On the other hand, there was only one person interviewed under the age of 35 that was interested in taking a passive role in the provider-patient relationship. It was also demonstrated that none of the people interviewed under the age of 35 (15 people) that we identified had "blind trust". Over the last 15 years, the concept of blind trust has diminished. The media and others have regularly shared "horror stories" about healthcare errors and omissions. Through this, consumers have increasingly come to understand that a medical degree does not automatically equate to competency. We expect that our doctors and other clinicians know what they are doing, our hospitals will care for us in a way that is correct and that the drug manufacturers are making drugs that are safe and effective. We trust in these things. That is what allows us to feel safe. One question that needs to be asked, are these things that we have just listed still true?

PwC in their annual megatrends document has stated that "the distrustful consumer" is one of the five megatrends facing healthcare. The article continues to describe how skepticism and distrust of traditional healthcare organizations has opened the door for non- traditional healthcare to compete. If healthcare providers and organizations want to regain trust issues such as greater convenience and access, more transparency, and improved outcomes are listed as necessary attributes

Let's take a minute and return to Seth. In our conversation, he spoke about the feeling of "being untethered." Webster's Dictionary defines the term untethered as unbound or disconnected. This is not how we want to feel when we are facing something unfamiliar or when we don't trust ourselves enough to handle a situation on our own. One way to address this feeling is to "have your person"- The television show Grey's Anatomy has coined the term" you are my person." We all want to have a person or as was stated above, "that teacher." Throughout most of history, your person was your primary care provider. The role of one's primary care provider is to help to address the feeling of being "untethered," to have someone that you have built a trusting relationship. This was the person that you saw for preventative care as well as when you were sick. Over the last 20 years the likelihood of a consumer having a relationship with a primary care provider has diminished. An Accenture 2019 Digital Health Consumer Survey had some disturbing data around the consumer/primary care provider relationship. The survey found that Gen Z and millennials are less likely to have a primary care doctor. That is not to say that they did not want one, but more often they stated they had yet to find one that they trusted.

This is different from baby boomers, Gen X and silent generation. It is not that they do not want one, it is just that many of them have not found someone that meets their needs (convenience) or desires (communication). In addition, this group stated that the availability of retail clinics and health services made a primary care provider unnecessary. A J.D. Power survey found that 48% of consumers had utilized at least one health service with a retail setting over the last year. (Ganguli, 2020). Many Gen Z say that they trust and align with alternative care such as acupuncturist or holistic care. (The Center for Consumer Engagement in Health Innovation, "In their Words: Consumers Vision for a Person-Centered Primary Care System." December 2019). This younger population stated that primary care doctors were not meeting their needs due to the lack of a trusting long - term relationship. They wanted more than a doctor with good credentials, they wanted someone empathetic to their needs and challenges as a patient. In addition, they were looking for providers that would help with physical, mental and social needs and they wanted a doctor that had understanding within the context of their cultural community.

There are a number of reasons that individuals give as to why they do not have a primary care provider. The responses vary:

a. They had primary care providers in the past but that the relationship was more of a "acquaintanceship,"
b. Relationships described as love/hate, aversion/hostility, enslavement, marriage of convenience. (NRC)
c. Democratization of healthcare through available information leading to perceived lack of need
d. The cost of seeing a primary care doctor
e. Their perceived lack of need for a primary care provider
f. Access and convenience of a primary care doctor (Ganguli, 2020)

Saul, a 42-year-old stated "having a doctor and having to go to see them is not like going to a flower shop. Going to the doctor is something I have to do; it is not something that I want to do. It does not bring me pleasure. If it is not convenient, costs too much or they are not pleasant to me. I just don't do it." He went on to say that he did have a primary provider for 6 years but then he moved. He has tried three doctors since and just "discarded" all three.

Our survey found that most of our participants (79%) had a primary care provider. And the relationship between having a PCP increased with age, while females were most likely to say they had a having a PCP.

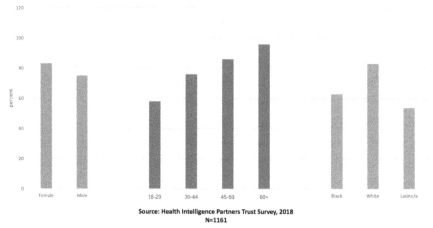

## I have a primary care provider
(i.e., a doctor I return to for regular check-ups or whenever I need basic medical care)

Source: Health Intelligence Partners Trust Survey, 2018
N=1161

# Age impact on having a primary care provider

| Generation | Percent |
|---|---|
| Silent Generation(1928-1945) | 85 |
| Baby Boomers (1946-1964) | 84 |
| Gen Xer(1965-1980) | 76 |
| Millennials(1981-1996) | 67 |
| Gen Z (1997-onward) | 55 |

Source: Accenture, 2019

Accenture 2019

It is not just the ability to identify one's primary care provider, it is also whether we utilize them. Ganguli in his 2020 paper discussed that the number of consumer visits to their primary care provider has been declining over the last 12 years. Over half of commercially insured consumers did not visit their primary care provider at all over a years period of time. The greatest decline was seen in younger adults, those without chronic conditions, and in lower socioeconomic areas. Again, our research skewed high in consumer utilization of their primary care provider in both number of office visits as well as other types of interactions. Out of the 79% of those that had a primary care provider, the majority of these people (78%) have seen their physician more than once or once a year.

Another area found to correlate with trust between the consumer and their providers is the length of the relationship. Trust tends to grow with time. The data from our study clearly showed this correlation. Nearly 80% of participants that responded to our survey have had their PCP for over 1 year with the largest single category of "more than 7 years" at 28%. Those who have had their doctor > 7 years, trust is higher. And for those who do not trust their doctor, it might be because they have had their doctor less than one year. Trust seems to dip in the middle categories between 3 and 7 years.

Unlike our data, Thomas Lee in his 2019 paper found that there was not a correlation between length of time of the relationship between the provider and the consumer. One reason for the discordance between Lee's data and ours may be tied to the differences in survey participants. Differences such as demographics and healthcare needs can create differences in responses associated with trust. When an consumer's health becomes more complicated, the trust between that individual and their provider tends to be more strained. In a healthcare environment where gatekeepers (e.g., utilization management and prior authorization) have a role, patients might feel their physician is to blame when a given procedure or treatment is denied or is very costly.

## Is There Trust?

The next question to delve into was whether the consumer/provider relationship is one built on trust. When asked people state that they trust their doctor that treats them but do not trust doctors in general. This comes back to interpersonal relationship versus societal relationship. It is hard to trust someone you do not know and have not had a relationship with. US ranked 24th in the percentage of people that stated that "all things considered, doctors in the US can be trusted. (Bendon RJ, Public Trust in Physicians. NEJM 2014; 37(17);1570-2.) In 1975, Gallup surveyed a population regarding their trust in the healthcare system. The survey showed that the population had a great deal of trust in healthcare. By 2015, Gallup found that only 37% of those surveyed had trust in the healthcare system. Although the survey found low levels of trust in the system, 73% trusted their doctor. In addition to trust of the provider in general, 56% say that their doctor "does a good job in providing diagnosis and treatment". Similar to other surveys, demographics such as age and race play a role in a consumer's level of trust in their doctor. Younger people, Blacks and Hispanics had lower level of trust(42%) in their providers to" provide an accurate diagnosis and correct treatment". (Pew)

Many have described the patient/physician relationship one of principle-agent relationship. Is the primary care provider, whether it is a physician or nurse practitioner, the agent of the patient, with the goal of maximizing the patient's health? If the physician as agent does not have the patient's best interest as their goal, who does? Overall, the Health Intelligence Partners survey found a high level of overall trust (90%) in one's primary care physician although it found differences in trust due to a number of demographic distinctions. One thing that we found consistently across all demographics was that the individuals trusted those doctors that put them first.

# I trust my primary care provider

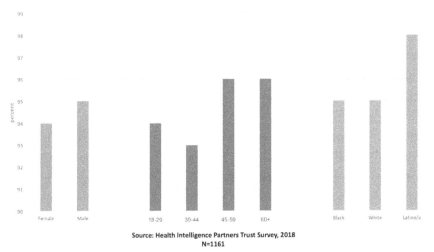

Source: Health Intelligence Partners Trust Survey, 2018
N=1161

In our earlier chart we saw that women were more likely to say they had a PCP; however, men were more likely to trust their PCP. Trust for those identifying a PCP, across gender, age and race was incredibly high.

> Susannah is a wonderful athlete. She shared with me that she had gone to the gym on Christmas Eve to work out prior to two days of festivities. Unfortunately, while working out, Susannah wrenched her back. Her back went into spasms that was causing significant pain. Susannah called her chiropractor and left a message. She did not expect to hear from him over the holiday. She shared her surprise when her phone rang early Christmas morning. It was her chiropractor apologizing for bothering her on the holiday and offered for her to come into the office. The caring and compassion of her doctor as well as putting her first has created a strong relationship and an atmosphere of trust. She shared that she now holds all of her providers to the level of care that she received from her chiropractor.

Our findings of high consumer trust are not unique. VHA and Deloitte through their healthcare data survey as far back as 2001 that most Americans trust their doctors. For the most part, this has not changed. 75% consider their doctors their most trustworthy source for healthcare information. (Healthcare 2001: A Strategic Assessment of the Healthcare Environment in the United States, AHA 2002.)

The Pew Research Center found in a 2019 study that 74% of those surveyed (4000 US Adults over the age of 18.), trust their provider. None the less, mistrust continues to be a significant issue. When the same cohort was asked whether they trusted their provider and believed that their doctors had their best interests:

- 57% stated all or most of the time
- 33% stated some of the time
- 9% stated only a little or none of the time

Further breakdown of the data found:

- 65% of seniors believe that their doctor had their best interest all or most of the time.
- 49% of younger adults believe that their doctor had their best interest all or most of the time.
- 73% of people "just look out for themselves and would try and take advantage of you if they could".
- 60% stated others "can't be trusted".

These metrics are compared across the backdrop of whether people, can be trusted. As you can see, trust of others is quite low in younger demographics.

- 18-29 years old stated that 40% of individuals can be trusted.
- 30-49 years old stated that 48% of individuals can be trusted.

- 50-64 years old stated that 57% of individuals can be trusted.
- 65+ years old stated that 71% of individuals can be trusted.

Our research did find that gender does have an impact on trust. Men are more likely to trust their physicians than women when they identify a specific PCP. Overall, however, men and women trusted their physician at a high level (men 88%, women 90% and for those who did not identify as a gender, 70%) This gender difference can be due to a number of factors including:

1. Men use healthcare less often. Frequently others prompt or push them to seek care. Men see healthcare as a tactical or financial arrangement. They are less likely to see healthcare through an emotional lens. However, when they identify as having a doctor, they appear to place more trust in them than women do.
2. Women interact with the healthcare system more than men. Women have a tendency to interact with healthcare through a relationship lens. They therefore stop using anyone that they do not trust and surround themselves with healthcare entities that they trust

## Gender Impact on Trust

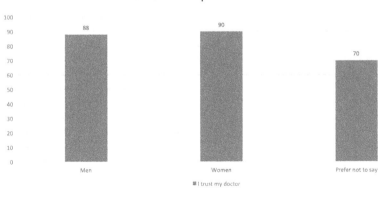

Source: Health Intelligence Partners Trust Survey, 2018
N=1161

We spoke about how socio-economic status can impact trust in general. This is also true when it comes to a consumer's trust in healthcare. Family financial difficulties impact trust, especially in very low-income situations. Those with family income under $30,000 are less trusting of their physician. Only 47% of low-income individuals state that their provider can be trusted. The data goes on to show that although one's financial position can have a significant influence on trust, the ability to afford healthcare is not the major driver. 63% of those with a higher income stated that they trust their healthcare provider. Although the percentage of trust in this higher socio-economic cohort, it is at an acceptable level when you consider the importance and impact that a healthcare provider can have on one's health.

## Income Impact on Trust

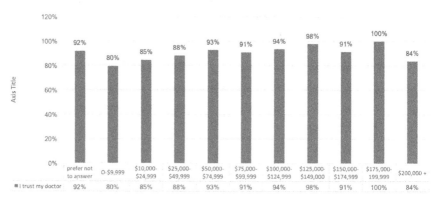

Source: Health Intelligence Partners Trust Survey, 2018
N=1161

# Age Impact on Trust

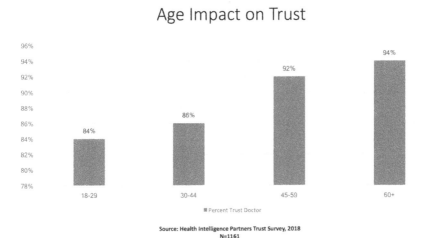

Source: Health Intelligence Partners Trust Survey, 2018
N=1161

One other consumer attribute associated with trust was that of care utilization. An example of this was found by the GE Camden Group. Their survey found that when aggregated, 81% of consumers were unsatisfied with their healthcare experience. This number seems to be higher than the results found by others. The more interesting data was found in the fact that in satisfaction and trust between those that utilized the healthcare system frequently (75% unsatisfied) versus those that were less frequent utilizers (48%) (GE Camden).

Although all those that we surveyed had high levels of trust, the geographic location of a respondent did seem to impact their level of trust. The West specifically reported the highest levels of trust in our survey.

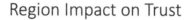

## Region Impact on Trust

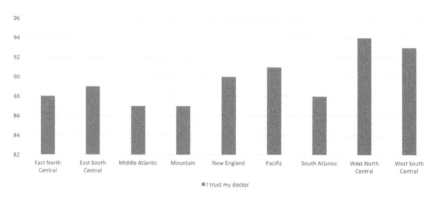

I trust my doctor

Source: Health Intelligence Partners Trust Survey, 2018
N=1161

## Issues Impacting Trust

What makes a person distrustful or dissatisfied with their healthcare? The literature and our surveys found a variety of reasons including access and convenience of care, being respected, cost and value, and aligned incentives. These issues matter to all demographics although vary to degree. One example of this is that younger individuals care more about convenience whereas older people care more about the quality of care. Let's take a few minutes and better understand a few of these findings.

1. Access and convenience- Human nature has found that if people believe that someone is available to them, they are more willing to trust. This is especially true in healthcare.
   a. Americans have a ferocious need for choice and control over the providers they see and the care that they receive regardless of whether it is necessary to good medicine. This unbridled desire of choice and access is not just found in healthcare. Next time you go to the grocery store, take a look at the peanut butter aisle. There are numerous choices we all can make as to what peanut butter

we put in grocery cart. That being said, lack of choice often creates suspicion and increases a lack of trust. As healthcare has become "more corporate", consumers are concerned that they are losing the access and control that they desire. When patients choose a doctor it often starts with trust.

> Jolene has 30 years of experience as a Healthcare executive. Earlier in her career she worked in a staff model HMO. She shared with us her experience when it came to consumer behavior within the HMO. "It was really interesting. This was a time with little or no patient out of pocket costs to see a primary care doctor. When they first joined the HMO, they came in often. They were afraid that they would not be seen. There had been so much bad press about the HMOs. Once they realized, that if they needed their doctor, they could get an appointment, they came in less often. Utilization became more appropriate. They needed to learn to trust their doctor and the system.

b. Convenience is often considered a form of access. While those surveyed had high praise for their providers, 78% stated that they were frustrated due to long waiting times. The 2019 Healthcare Consumer Trends Report by NRC Health interviewed 1,000,000 individuals. The data was insightful. 80% of those surveyed stated that they would change providers in order to get convenience and access that they desired. (NRC). Gen Z consumers felt that convenience and affordability were important aspects in choosing a trusting provider

c. We have seen an increasing number of alternative care sites and organizations over the last several years. Many of these care venues have arisen due to access and convenience challenges. Studies have shown that 69% of consumers still prefer their own provider over urgent care (29%) and (10%) retail care sites. (Health Care Consumer Trust Survey, Bright MD, 2019)

| Who Do You Trust With to Provide Your Healthcare | Percent |
|---|---|
| Your health care system or provider | 66.7 |
| Other Healthcare providers or systems | 54.1 |
| Stand alone urgent care centers | 29.3 |
| Health Insurance Plan | 26.3 |
| Retailer (CVS, Walmart) | 9.9 |
| Web-based care | 7.1 |
| Technology Company (Google, Apple) | 4.4 |

Source: Healthcare Consumer Trust Survey, Bright MD, 2019

# The Importance of Earning Loyalty

Will switch providers for "convenience factors"

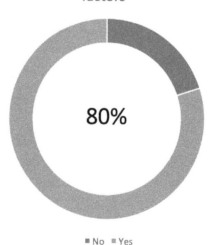

80%

■ No  ■ Yes

**Source: 2019 Healthcare Consumer Trend Report, NRC Healthcare**

2. Feeling "seen" and respected- We all look to be respected. Think about a time when you felt disrespected by someone. Did you want to spend time with that person or have a relationship with them? Probably not. It is difficult to trust someone if you sense a lack of respect.

   a. Gen Z consumers state that if their doctor does not listen to them and actively engage with them, they will fire them.

   b. A subset of consumers sees their doctors as being driven by profit with little time to listen to or focus on them. Interestingly, it did not matter whether the provider was part of a for profit or non-for-profit organization.

   c. A survey done by NRC found that 87% of patients found their providers to be courteous and respectful. They went on to say that this was not the case with the providers staff, where only 33% of those asked felt respected. This lack of respect has impacted the relationship and trust both with their doctor and in the system. (NRC)

      > Gordie is a 29 year- old who spoke to us about an experience he had in a provider's office. "I signed in at the front desk at the doctor's office. The man behind the desk did not look up or acknowledge my presence. After a few minutes I went back up to the front desk and verbally let the gentleman know that I had arrived. The response from the receptionist was "what do you want, a tickertape parade." I was both angry and embarrassed. When I shared the episode with my doctor, he told me to just ignore the receptionist as it was just meant to be funny. I never went back to that doctor. Neither he nor his staff respected me. "

   d. "Nothing about me, without me" has become a slogan utilized by a number of patient advocacy groups. Asymmetry in knowledge often brings lack of trust between the consumer and their provider. The inequality of knowledge often leads to the feeling of an unequal relationship. Interestingly one area where the patient has more knowledge than the provider is in their desires, goals and the actions that they take after they leave the doctor's office. The patient often decides they cannot share this information as they feel that it will reduce the doctor's trust in them and that the doctor will think that they do not trust the doctor.

e.  A Deloitte study found that 58% of consumers said that they were either very likely or likely to disagree with their doctors when an issue arises. Unfortunately, many consumers stated that their doctor seemed to not hear them when they voiced their concerns.

f.  As providers are practicing "population health" patients have become concerned that the doctor is looking at the population and not the patient in front of them.

3.  Aligned incentives -Misaligned goals create an atmosphere where it is difficult to form or maintain a trusting relationship. Conflict of interest, due to cost or relationship issues can also impact trust. Today's healthcare system contains areas of concern for about whether the provider is looking out for the consumers interest or their own. A number of those had a similar question regarding who is on their side and fighting for them. As we discussed during the definitions part of the book, in order to trust someone, there needs to be belief that the other person or entity has aligned interests and is willing to put your goals and desires before theirs. This study shows that consumers rarely believe that when it comes to healthcare costs, those within the healthcare industry have their best interests in mind.

a.  20% of Gen Z consumers state that they have not found a doctor that meets their needs or that they trust to put their needs first. (Accenture Digital Health consumer survey).

b.  Consumers and the provider are involved in a form of a

principal-agent contractual relationship. Many patients have questioned whether the provider is the agent of the consumer or is the provider an agent of another such as the health plan or the health system. There is concern that the physician is more focused of meeting the needs and the goals of others than themselves, whether it be the employer as the payer, the health plan as the adjudicator and the person that pays the doctor, the hospital where the doctor must maintain admitting privileges (and most recently may be the payer) or the pharmaceutical company in the case of a clinical trial.

c.  Many consumers feel that providers have given up the decision making that is necessary in caring for them.

> Sim went to see his provider in order to get a prescription refill for a medication that he had been on for several years for his migraine headaches. His doctor shared with him that he could not prescribe the medication that had been working for him due to formulary constraints. "Who is my doctor, Dr Jones or the insurance company? Shame on him." He went on to share that this realization created a loss in trust for Dr Jones.

There are a number of reasons that patients have lost confidence in the system. The Pew study found that in fact, physicians are often not open and honest with their patients about conflict of interest.

- 15% are transparent about conflict of interest all or most of the time
- 50% are transparent about conflict of interest some of the time
- 33% are transparent about conflict of interest little or none of the time

This is very different from historical feelings of patients when they felt that there were not others that were "involved or in the middle of their relationship" with their doctor.

    d. There has been a great deal of press regarding financial relationships between physicians and pharmaceutical companies. A study by Grande and his co- authors found that 55% of patients believed that their doctor received gifts from the drug companies that impacted prescribing habits. This was more common in younger patients and those of higher socio-economic status

4. Quality of Care and Cost- All of us want the best care possible. In addition, we want our care to be affordable. The combination of cost and quality point to the value that the consumer believes that they are getting. Value has become an important attribute across society. Just as a consumer looks for value in things such as cars and meals, they expect value in their healthcare as well.

    a. Although 55% of Generation Z consumers (born after 1997) have a primary care provider, one third of them are dissatisfied with the treatment effectiveness that they have received. (Accenture Digital Health consumer survey).

    b. 41% of Gen Z consumers are dissatisfied with the cost of their care and the lack of transparency of the cost. (Accenture Digital Health Consumer Survey).

5. Communication- what we say and how we say it.

> Lila is an older woman that went to see a specialist for an acute medical problem. She had not seen this physician in the past. At the end of the visit the physician gave her a DVD and paper document with information on how to address her symptoms. "L" became very frustrated because the two documents were difficult to understand and contradicted each other. She was unsure if the doctor had not reviewed the two resources and therefore did not know that they were not consistent or if he did

not know which treatment was correct. Lila shared her frustration and lack of trust due to the situation

## Do provider differences matter when it comes to trust?

During our conversations with consumers regarding trust in primary care providers, we identified two additional interesting factors. The first focuses on provider employment status. Although patients state that they trust their physicians, they do not necessarily trust hospitals, health systems, health insurers or the healthcare industry as a whole. One of the questions that we will have to watch closely will be now that employed physicians outnumber independent doctors, will this impact trust. As of June of 2019, 47.7% of physicians are employed by larger organizations. (Medical Economics, June 10, 2019, page 4)

Early data on this issue are concerning. Consumers have been found to have greater trust in providers that were self-employed versus those employed by health insurers or health systems. Consumers felt that those that were employed had greater issues in regard to conflict of interest than those that were independent.

Contractually, the patient and the provider are involved in a principal-agent relationship. Many patients have questioned whether the provider is the agent or is the physician an agent of another such as the health plan or the health system. There is concern that the physician is more focused of meeting the needs and the goals of others than themselves, whether it is the employer as the payer, the health plan as the adjudicator and the person that pays the doctor, the hospital where the doctor must maintain admitting privileges (and most recently may be the payer) or the pharmaceutical company in the case of a clinical trial.

Our data seems to concur with others that found the same sentiment in those that they surveyed. One example of this is that of LUGPA, an organization that represents Urology Practitioners in the United

States. In a survey conducted December 3, 2018, 65% of individuals surveyed stated that they trust independent providers over those employed by a hospital. This differentiation of trust in practitioners due to the evolving employment model creates a challenge as more providers are employed by healthcare organizations.

The second factor was the difference in trust in primary care providers and specialists. As stated, up until the early 1980s it was customary for the consumer to have a long -term relationship with one provider, their primary care doctor. It was not until the middle of the 20th century that doctors began to specialize. By 2015, only 33% of those with a medical degree were primary care doctors with the remainder becoming specialists or subspecialists. (Dalen J. Where Have the Generalists Gone? The American Journal of Medicine, 130(7), July 2017) The reasons for the decrease in primary care provider utilization with the associated increase in specialty provider utilization can be partially attributed to the increasing number of individuals with chronic health conditions, the increasing need for specialty care in order to address these conditions and the increasing use of specialty providers over primary care to address this type of care.

> Josephine is a 71 -year -old woman with diabetes and heart disease. She shared with us her frustration in "juggling" all the information that she gets from her doctors. "I have five doctors and am on nine medicines. It is not unusual that the doctors give me advice or information that conflicts. It is confusing and makes me angry. I don't think that they talk to each other. How am I supposed to know who is right, who is wrong and who to trust? I just get mad and don't know who to trust. When I get mad enough, I don't do what any of them say.

There is an additional area of provider specialist that has created challenges in the provider/consumer trust equation, the hospitalist. Historically, when patients were admitted to the hospital, their primary care doctor or the specialist that was caring for them in an outpatient setting remained their doctors during their hospital stay. During the 1990s we began to see the use of hospitalists, physicians that cared for the patient during their hospital stay. In most cases, there was no previous interactions between these providers and the patient. This change may make sense from a clinical viewpoint, but at the same time has created both confusion and a lack of trust. During our interviews, over 50% of the people we spoke to said that they had trust challenges with the hospitalists that they or their family member had dealt with during a hospital stay. "They do not know me, how do they know what I want or need," "When I was in the hospital, I saw different hospital doctors every day.

There was no consistency. This also meant that I had to keep answering the same questions." "who the hell is in charge of my care. You keep telling me I should have a primary doctor and then when I am at my sickest, you take that doctor away from me and give me a stranger. This is stupid."

> Samantha was an otherwise healthy senior. She unfortunately found herself in the emergency room with shortness of breath. The initial healthcare team that treated her, diagnosed a pneumonia and began treatment. Samantha was told that she would be staying overnight in the hospital due to her age, her presenting symptoms and potential drug side effects. Over Samantha's time in the emergency room, there was a shift change. The new clinical team told Samantha that she would be going home after finishing her initial antibiotic dosages. When asked why the change in plans, Samantha was told that it was normal protocol. When the family became involved and a conversation occurred with the emergency room team, it became evident that there was a limited amount of transition conversation that had occurred. This conflicting plan created a lack of trust by both Samantha and her family.

Our research found that there are trust differences between primary care providers and specialists. At a high level it was found that the compassion portion attached to consumer/provider trust weighed much greater for the relationship with the primary care provider whereas the competence portion was more heavily weighted for specialists. The logic of this makes sense. People that are seeing a specialist tend to have more serious medical problems and therefore the consumer needs to trust these providers to cure or significantly improve the medical condition that brought the consumer to the specialist in the first place.

Again, we need to remember overall consumer trust in providers is high. Most people that we spoke to trust their provider and felt their doctors did have their best interest. Yes, there are things that providers can continue to do to maintain trust or improve trust. In the third section of the book, we will offer recommendations for addressing some 'trust resets."

## Consumer Trust in the Science and Scientists

Science is what healthcare is based on. Prevention, treatment and cure of a consumer's medical problems all take their cues from what science and scientists find in the evidence. In order to trust those that directly or indirectly care for us, we as consumers need to trust that science that is the basis for our care. The question is do consumers trust scientists and inventors? The answer is yes and no. This is not a new question. Let's take a moment and look at the history of human vaccines. Some would say that vaccinations are one of the most significant achievements in public health. Others such as the Anti-vaccination Leagues in the United States and England would strongly disagree. As far back as the late 1800s with the discovery of the smallpox vaccine, a group of individuals did not trust the inventors of the smallpox vaccine nor the vaccine itself. This debate continues today. 55% stated that they trust medical scientists' and physicians' information regarding vaccines by giving full information on the impact of vaccines for their families and friends. As you can see, the consumers surveyed were less trusting of other stakeholders when it comes to vaccine information. Only 13% trust the pharmaceutical manufacturers of vaccines to provide strong scientific advice. Many in the "distrust the manufacturer" belief set feel that the manufacturers care more about making money than helping consumers. It is unclear as to whether this lack of trust is based on religious, spiritual, political or philosophical terms. Individuals with a greater knowledge of science, higher education and in higher socio-economic status are more trusting of the vaccines. The study also found that Blacks tended to be less trusting of the vaccines and believed that there was greater risk to the vaccines that were not disclosed. (Funk, 2017)

# Most Americans say medical scientists should have a major policy role on vaccine issues

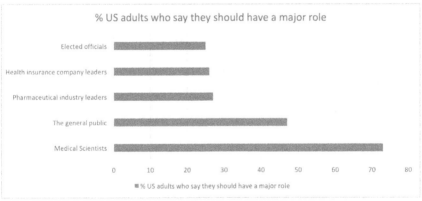

**Source: Pew, From Washington Post, 2017**

Pew Research Center has followed consumer trust in the scientific community since 1973. The good news is that confidence in science and scientists has remained relatively stable over that time with 95% of those surveyed stating that scientists are "helping to solve challenging problems." (Trust and Confidence at the Interfaces of the Life Sciences and Society: Does the Public Trust Science? National Academies of

Sciences, Engineering and Medicine. 2015) Unfortunately, there are actions that challenge this trust. One example of this is when a medication previously found to be safe is later found to have significant side effects. Vioxx was a very popular nonsteroidal anti-inflammatory used for a number of health conditions. In 2004, five years after entering the market, Vioxx was removed from the market due to the increased risk of heart attacks. The effect of this medication withdrawal from the market increased distrust in similar medications and a 30% decrease in the use of them. A second example of how the actions of a few scientists have impacted science and scientists more broadly is based on questions regarding the credibility of research. On several occasions over the last few years academic papers have been based on exaggerated, false or misleading data. In other cases, we find that the authors of articles are being published by scientists that have financially based conflicts of interest. Consumer's trust is chipped away each time we learn that scientific journals are ethically challenged.

## Provide Fair and Accurate Statements and Advice

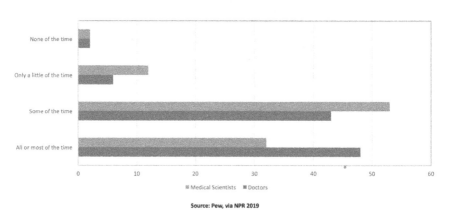

Source: Pew, via NPR 2019

Scientists working in healthcare, nutrition and the environment all face very different levels of trust over the last few years. The need for trust in both science and scientists is imperative as consumers look to innovation in healthcare to improve health. A 2019 Pew Research study found that overall, the public's trust in scientists has been increasing since 2016. This improvement of trust comes at a time when trust in science and scientists has been impacted due to significant ideological differences and a world-wide pandemic. How these factors will impact trust in science and scientists in the long term has yet to be determined.

## The Consumer and the Health Care Organizations

Healthcare has changed significantly since the 1980s. Prior to that time there were three dominant stakeholders associated with healthcare; the consumer, the doctor and the hospital. Most consumers rarely interacted with hospitals and when they did, they still saw the hospital as an extension of their relationship with their doctor. Over the last 40 years, the number of stakeholders within the healthcare environment have expanded.

These changes have created strain in trust between the patient and much of the healthcare system. This complex matrix of stakeholders includes both individuals and organizations. As we talked about earlier in the book, there is a difference in trust between consumers and other individuals versus trust between an individual and an organization. This mix of individuals versus organizations in healthcare creates a trust dichotomy. It is much easier to trust a person than a "thing."

> "You can't look an organization in the eye"
> Elan, 24-year-old male.

This is not to say that hospitals, health systems and health insurance companies are not trusted by the healthcare consumer. At a high level many health systems do have the trust of their patients although less than the individual healthcare provider. When asked, patients want more than excellent care from the health system, they want to know that the system is "on their side" and cares about them. They are looking for costs that they can afford and convenience that is similar to what they receive in other areas within society. Over the last several years there has been an increase in focus on value within healthcare. We asked several of those that we spoke to about their feelings on value in healthcare. We received a number of interesting comments. The one thing that all the individuals agreed upon is that the conversation on value does not increase trust in the consumer.

1. "No one asked me. Were patients included in the conversation"
2. "Value to who? I bet the value goes to the CEO of the Health Plan and the doctor"
3. " I don't know how to evaluate whether the care I get has value. I would assume I need it because my doctor ordered it"

The cost of healthcare for the consumer continually comes up as a determinant in the issue of trust. Direct financial interactions are a common occurrence between the consumer and providers as well as others such as health plans, hospitals and pharmacies. Over the last several years, consumers are being asked to take on a greater cost burden. The increased cost responsibility of the consumer is often a barrier to access. This issue has created feelings of frustration and anger leading to a decrease in trust in the system. This frustration is magnified by the complex financial arrangements that occur between the multitude of stakeholders within the healthcare system. The consumer hears about financial arrangements between hospitals, insurance companies, drug manufacturers, pharmacies and others through the press and other information outlets. It is common for consumers to misunderstand these relationships due to the complexity as well as the secrecy and lack of transparency that shrouds them. Even when there are no financial relationships between the stakeholders, many patients believe that they exist.

Our survey respondents trust their hospital to give them correct information much more than their insurance company or their health system. In general, we found that older age groups have a greater trust in healthcare as a whole but lag behind younger adults, when it comes to trusting information received from hospital sources.

# I trust my hospital with my healthcare information

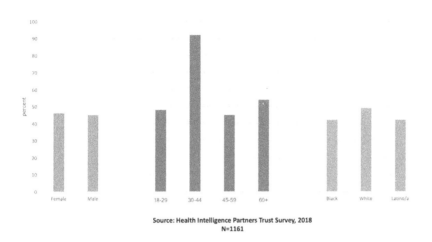

**Source: Health Intelligence Partners Trust Survey, 2018**
**N=1161**

## I trust the healthcare system with my healthcare information

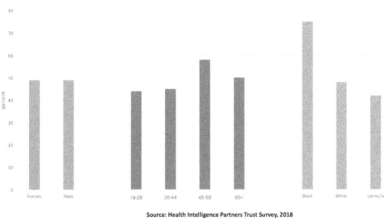

**Source: Health Intelligence Partners Trust Survey, 2018**
**N=1161**

## I trust my insurer with my healthcare information

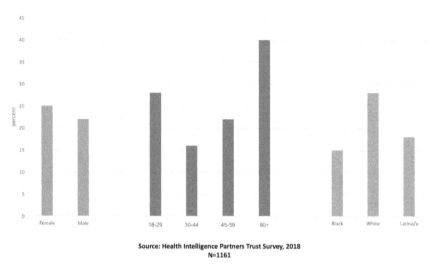

Source: Health Intelligence Partners Trust Survey, 2018
N=1161

Andre is a 41 -year- old male that shared his feelings about transparency in healthcare costs. "I was always taught that if you are not willing to share information, you are hiding something. I don't understand why hospitals don't want to share what my care is going to cost me. I am asked by my employer and my health insurance to make good decisions. I don't know how to do this unless you tell me how much I am going to spend. I am not sure who is hiding what but clearly the hospital is hiding something.... Why should I trust an organization that is not being honest with me?"

A number of individuals felt that their health care insurance and health systems were primarily focused on "making money." There has been a lot of talk about patients feeling that profit comes before of people with pharma, providers (beyond their own) and insurance. When asked if it made a difference whether the organization that was not - for- profit versus those that were for- profit we found little difference. In fact, very few individuals knew whether the hospitals that they or their family used and the companies that they were insured by were for profit or not for profit. Most assumed all these health care entities were for profit. The media often points out these types of financial arrangements are often focused on money and profit. The bad behavior of a few have created a distrust of many.

> When talking with John, he articulated this difference well. He spoke about a situation where he went to see his doctor about a medical problem he was having. His neighbor had recently had a similar problem and had a large battery of tests to diagnose the issue. After speaking with John, his doctor made a diagnosis. No tests were needed to reach this answer. John shared with us that he trusted his doctor's knowledge and therefore was willing to accept the diagnosis without the tests that his neighbor had received. John went on to share with us that if he had to rely on the healthcare system, John would have pushed for the tests. "My doctor I trust, the healthcare system I do not trust. All the system wants to do is save money

A recent Pew survey of healthcare consumers asked:

How much do you trust the following to keep costs low?

1. Federal Government:
   47% stated not much/not at all

2. Providers:
   52% stated not much/not at all

3. Private Insurance
   68% stated not much/not at all

4. Pharmaceutical industry
   75% stated not much/not at all

## Health Plans

Boulware's study of 118 individuals found that study participants trusted physicians and hospitals more than Health Insurance Plans. Interestingly, when study participants were broken down by race it was found that African American study participants were more likely to trust their Health Insurance Plan than their doctors or hospitals. Again, this most likely aligns to concerns over real or perceived discrimination or racism either directly or passed down through historical experience of others.

For healthcare treatment/advice do you trust any of the following (check all that apply)

| Answer | Percent (rounded to nearest 2 digit | N |
|---|---|---|
| My doctor | 89 | 952 |
| My friend | 36 | 275 |
| My pharmacist/pharmacy | 58 | 616 |
| The pharmaceutical manufacturer / maker of medicines that you may take | 9 | 93 |
| My urgent care facility, ED, or retail health clinic (e.g. CVS, Walgreens | 38 | 401 |
| My hospital | 47 | 500 |
| Online, internet or tele-health | 20 | 212 |
| Health insurance provider (e.g. United, BCBS, Aetna) | 13 | 141 |

Source: Health Intelligence Partners Trust Survey, 2018
N=1161

The Pew Foundation found that people do not go to their insurers for decisions for a number or reasons including that they do not feel that the insurance company has their best interests.

Earlier in the book we discussed the importance of trust in creating a lasting and loyal relationship. This has been found to be true whether we are discussing consumer trust in the provider, hospital system, health insurance Company, or pharmacy. NRC and others that studied the impact on trust have found that this increasing lack of trust across healthcare has created declines in loyalty. (NRC)

LUGPA released a national survey of 1192 patients. Over 60% stated that they were worried about the mergers and acquisitions of doctor' groups and hospitals. Additionally, 25% stated that this growth was a threat to their health. Overall, those surveyed stated that they trusted smaller organizations such as independent physicians more than those that were working for hospitals. (65%). LIGPA is a nonprofit urology trade association.

Frustration surrounding treatment and coverage decisions has been identified as the largest trust buster. In addition to these utilization management issues, there are two additional areas that consumers often identify as dissatisfiers that lead to distrust. The first focuses on the provider network associated with the health plan. Consumers historically chose their providers through word of mouth and recommendations from others that they trusted. Many of the health insurance plans no longer offer this freedom of choice. Although this closed provider panel was found as far back as the Pierce County Medical Group, The Baylor Model for teachers in Texas and in Kaiser, it was not the prominent model for many years. Consumers were able to see who they chose without limitations. The HMO Act of 1973 brought the return of the provider network model. In the case of HMOs, the provider network was a closed model. In order to have your services paid for, you had to see a doctor within the insurance company's network. Outside of the HMO model of insurance, the provider network was often broader with some providers being preferred and others not. Consumers paid less to see the preferred providers. Unfortunately, there was often no explanation as to why one provider was preferred over another. Most recently, we have seen a return to a closed provider model with "narrow networks." This has created great frustration and increased levels of distrust by consumers.

The second area that creates high levels of distrust is in the administrative inefficiencies of a health plan. How many times have you been left on hold? How many times have you been given conflicting answers by your health plan?

Maria is a 52- year -old woman that works in a large retail setting. She has worked in the service industry for 27 years. "If I treated the public the way my health plan treats me, I would have been fired years ago. I think that they do it on purpose. They make it really hard and unpleasant when we call them, because they don't want us to call. When we do call them, they are rude, uncaring and never really answer the question we are asking. They hope we will just give up. My insurance told me that I had to call to get permission to have an x-ray that my doctor ordered. I did just what they told me to do. When I called them, they told me that maybe it would be covered. That the insurance company would decide after I had my test. If they could not ok it, why do I have to call them. Waste of my time and waste of their time. Stupid."

Provider Networks and administrative inefficiencies as also found to be trust busters between providers and health plans. When actions are universally disliked and create trust barriers across a number of stakeholders, one would conclude that the system needs to be revised.

## Hospitals and Hospital Systems

Patients trust in hospitals has also taken a hit over the last 30 years. Most of us do not like going to the hospital but once we were sent there, we trusted the hospital to be competent and look out for our best interests. In 1976, Michael Jellinik wrote a paper that discussed the erosion of trust by patients in large medical centers. The size of these hospitals as well as lack of personal attention was found to be the greatest factor.

Gillian, a 61- year -old woman shared her feelings about hospitals. I want to trust hospitals because I have to put my life in their hands. The problem is that there is not "a person" that is responsible. I never know where to turn when there is a problem. "I was in a car accident and was hospitalized for 4 days. Technically, the care was fine. Unfortunately, there were two incidents that were very disturbing on the personal front. I wanted to talk to someone about this. I asked three times to speak with someone while I was in the hospital. No one came to speak with me. I then made two additional attempts via telephone once I got home. Again, no response. I know that they are busy, but it just felt like no one cared."

Gillian and others like her are not looking to understand how the hospitals processes work. What they are looking for is compassion and care. They are also looking for information and to be heard. Having to go the hospital can be a frightening experience. We are ill, potentially in pain and outside of our normal routine.

In 2006, The Cleveland Clinic hired Dr. Bridget Duffy to be the organizations first Chief Experience Officer. Dr Duffy, an internal medicine physician is considered the founder of the patient experience movement. When asked whether she trusts hospitals, she stated that for the most part hospitals are transactional. "It is up to the consumer to navigate the system." During her time at Cleveland Clinic, she looked to address this issue of navigation. She worked to create an experience where the consumer was "guided through their entire journey." When talking with Dr. Duffy, you get the sense that the patient experience is something that she is passionate about. She talks about the importance of an empathetic encounter and how that experience creates both trust and better healthcare outcomes. The patient experience movement has increased within hospitals and hospital systems over the last 10 years. In 2006, The Centers for Medicare and Medicaid Services (CMS) developed the Hospital Consumer Assessment of Healthcare Providers and Systems (HCAHPS) survey. In 2008 these scores were made available to the public. It is the goal of CMS and others that these data help consumers to identify important quality metrics and choose hospitals and hospital systems that they can trust.

Trust is an important factor when we find ourselves in a vulnerable position. There are few times in which we are more vulnerable than when we need hospitalization. Having one's family member or themselves needing a hospital requires trust. It is an emotional time. There are times that trust is lost due to the high emotions associated with serious illness.

> Florio is a 39 -year- old male. Florio shared a story of his loss in trust of a large university- based hospital in his hometown. Over an eight- year period both my mother and my sister died in the same hospital. Maybe it was the hospitals fault and maybe it wasn't. I just know that I really do not want any other family members to go to that hospital. No one comes out alive."

## Consumer Trust in their Employers

The Edelman Trust Survey of 2019 found that 75% of those surveyed felt that their employer was a "trusted relationship" whereas businesses in general was only found to have a 56% trust level. Like the issue with doctors (medicine is not to be trusted but my doctor is), this is also true with employers. Approximately fifty percent of Americans receive their health insurance through their employer. How do individuals feel about their employers regarding their health benefits? In general, employees are satisfied with their healthcare benefits. A 2018 survey found that over 70% of employers were "generally satisfied." Seventy five percent felt that their employer health plan helps them with most of their medical costs. (AHIP Value of Employer Provided Coverage Survey, February 2018).

As the United States and the world battle COVID 19, the role of employers and the consumers trust regarding preparedness to address their health and safety has been identified by several surveys. An updated Edelman Trust Survey done in March of 2020 found that consumers trust employers more than government to educate and support them during the pandemic. Those surveyed stated that the most credible source of information was the employer.

Even with high levels of satisfaction and trust, concerns remain. Over the last several years, employers have increased employee out of pocket responsibility of healthcare costs. The increase of high deductible health insurance plan designs and other plan designs that include higher co-pay and co-insurance resulting in increased financial and decision-making responsibility on the consumer has placed an increasing strain on the employee-employer relationship. The trust relationship between a consumer and their employer is challenged.

## Consumers and data sharing

The last 20 years has created an environment where data is more abundant and more necessary. One area of importance regarding trust between the consumer and the various stakeholders in healthcare is the sharing of information. Think about the last time you went to your doctor. The likelihood is that the conversation that ensued included sharing information about your health. It may also have included concerns and questions that you had. Trust between a consumer and their provider allows for greater information sharing. Trust allows us to be vulnerable and believe that our providers will use the data to help us. As science and technology have advanced, so has the amount of information that can be collected by both the consumer and the healthcare system. Consumers are willing to share their medical data under certain circumstances. Our data has shown that consumers share their data with those that they know; the healthcare provider including their primary care provider or health specialist, their nurse and their pharmacists. Trust is directly aligned with relationships. As more relationships are short term, trust seems to go down and the willingness to share personal information decreases. Consumers also are willing to share information with friends and family. Interestingly, many consumers were willing to share information with friends more than family. The reasons for this disparity between friends and family is due to the concern over familial judgment regardless if the consumer is young or older.

> Aletha is 25- year- old. When asked about sharing her health care information she laughed and said "I am willing to share my information with anyone except my parents. I share everything with my friends. My friends are the people I turn to when I need help. I love my parents but I there are lots of things that I don't share with them."

> Donald is an 83-year-old. His comments regarding the sharing of health information with friends was similar to Aletha's. "I have no problem talking about my medical problems with my friends. Most of them are going through the same things that I am. It is not something we talk about at the golf course but if I needed to, I would tell my buddies. Will I tell my kids, no way? They will put me in one of those homes. Without my independence, I have no life."

Whereas many consumers are comfortable sharing health data and information with other individuals, only about 50% were willing to share information with organizations. Consumers are less likely to share their health information with healthcare organizations such as hospitals, health plans and governmental organizations. The reasons for this are consistent across our research as well as the research of other organizations. Almost universally, consumers stated that their reticence in sharing health data and information is due to the lack of trust in how the data will be used.

> Stanos a 51-year-old, is willing to share his health information with his friends like Aletha and Donald, Stanos also shares his health issues and concerns with his son and daughter in law. "I have nothing to hide, they are family." When asked about sharing his information with his health plan, Stanos smiled. "I

don't trust the insurance companies. They are always finding ways to withhold coverage. If I tell them what is wrong with me or share other information, they will probably take away my medical coverage."

Stanos was not alone in these feelings. Only one in five individuals were willing to share their information with health insurance organizations. Almost universally, trust in sharing personal health information with governmental agencies was low. This aligned more broadly with individuals trust in the government.

Gender has been found to make a difference in consumers trust patterns. Although Aletha and Donald were of different gender and ages, they agreed on who they were willing to share their medical information with. Although Donald has no difficulty sharing his information with his "buddies," it was more theoretical whereas Aletha talked about how she and her friends often talk about their health issues such as weight and their aches and pains. This difference in sharing is not due to trust but due to differences in relationship types that men and women form. Men's friendships are more functional and less emotional whereas women form friendships that more intimate and supportive.

In addition to gender, age also has been shown to factor into one's trust patterns. Older individuals are more likely to share information with their doctors. It is common that information sharing is broader than those of younger ages, especially those under 45 years old. Younger consumers tend to share only that which they feel is pertinent to the issue that they are seeking care for. This is often due to the longitudinal relationship that has been formed between older consumers and their healthcare provider. Another area of trust and healthcare information sharing that aligns with age is that of social media and on-line sharing of health information. Although there was no population that had a significant level of trust sharing information over the internet, those under 29 years old were more willing to do so than those over 29.

One other interesting trust factor that we found is that younger consumers under the age of 29 and those over 65 people show more altruism towards helping society in health and are willing to share their information and data in order to achieve this.

These groups have articulated that the value of their health data outweighs any trust issues that they may have. They feel that their health data can help to "provide better care for myself and others.

## If you gave someone information about your health or illnesses, who would you trust it with? (check all that apply)

| Answer | Percent (rounded to nearest 2 digits) | N |
|---|---|---|
| My doctor | 92 | 957 |
| My friends/family | 41 | 422 |
| My pharmacist/pharmacy | 42 | 440 |
| The drug manufacturer of my medicines | 4.2 | 42 |
| My hospital | 50 | 517 |
| Online questions on the internet or telehealth) | 7.2 | 76 |
| Health Insurance provider (e.g., United, BCBS, Aetna) | 21 | 217 |
| Government | 5.1 | 54 |

Source: Health Intelligence Partners Trust Survey, 2018
N=1161

| Who do you trust with your healthcare information? | Percent |
|---|---|
| Your healthcare system or provider | 68.9 |
| Other healthcare providers or systems | 21.8 |
| Stand alone urgent care centers | 49.7 |
| Retailer (CVS, Walmart) | 16.5 |
| Web-based care | 8.0 |
| Technology Company (Apple, Google) | 8.3 |

Source: Healthcare Consumer Trust Survey, Bright MD, 2019

## Consumer Trust in the Government

Public trust in government is at an all -time low. According to Pew Research, only 17% of Americans say that they trust the government to do what is right. This contrasts with 1958 when Pew began measuring public trust in government. This paucity of trust is similar across generational as well as racial and ethnic groups. (Public Trust in Government, 1958-2019 Pew Research Center, April 11, 2019). With this as a backdrop, how does government fair regarding their impact on health and healthcare?

The question as to whether healthcare is a right or a privilege has been an on-going conversation. There is a great deal of disagreement as regards this issue. Many individuals especially young adults feel that healthcare and education are rights that should be readily available through governmental systems for all citizens. When they hear from certain governmental institutions that decide that it is not a right, they lose trust. A second question that is often asked focuses on government's role in health and healthcare. The United States government has played a significant role in healthcare since 1965 with the launch of Medicare and Medicaid. Through both coverage, governmental agencies, policy and legislative action, the United States government has a significant impact on both consumers and healthcare organizations. At the same time, we find that less than 50% of Americans trust the government when it comes to their health. (McPhillips Deidre, Majority of Americans Don't Trust Government with their Health. U.S. New and World Report. March 26, 2020)

## The Provider and Trust
### THE PROVIDER AS A HUMAN

> For us to really address the issue of trust across healthcare, all stakeholders have to have trust as a value (Richard Baron, MD)

As we begin the conversation about the healthcare provider, we need to remember providers are human. The same role that demographics and other traits have on consumers are found in providers as well. Biases, beliefs, communication styles and other behaviors that we discussed earlier come to play in regard to trust and the healthcare provider.

Bias, both implicit and explicit, can be initiated by one party to another. Providers not only carry their own biases and beliefs with them, they are also the recipient of other's biases and beliefs. Similar to other professions, healthcare has become increasingly diverse in its racial, gender and cultural makeup. Fifty-one percent of providers in the US are non-Caucasion, 28% are foreign born and 34% are women. This increase in diverse workforce brings with it a great deal of value. Finnegan and others have talked about the positive impact that ethnic and racial provider/patient concurrence can have on trust. (Finnegan J.) Unfortunately, it has also brought with it an increase in racist activity both propagated by providers and against healthcare providers. The NRC 2019 Consumer Trend Report identified a trend of increasing incidence of providers being verbally demeaned by their patients. This survey found that in between the patient and the provider, 59% of physicians reported being demeaned by a patient within the last 5 years. (NRC, 2019) "From the N-word to catcalls, physicians talk about demeaning behavior from biased patients. (Fierce Healthcare, Oct, 2019; JAMA Internal Medicine, Oct. 2019.) Providers are beginning to speak up about the increasing incidence of verbally and physically abusive behavior by their patients. This behavior has been shown to occur across race, gender, religion, sexual orientation and culture. A study performed at the University of California, which included 50 participants, discussed the emotional impact and the trust degredation of these interactions. Participants spoke of feelings of betrayal, emotional pain, confusion, reduction in well-being and negative impact in their trust of patients.

In addition to these human traits and characteristics, the education and indoctrination of providers must be understood as these experiences also have an impact on issues associated with trust. To become a physician takes years of education within a very competitive atmosphere. It is not unusual for students in a first- year medical school to be told to "look to the left and look to the right." They are then told that one of you will not make it through medical school to be a doctor. This statement creates a very competitive environment. It also brings about a situation in which those that do graduate often find themselves having a greater sense of self. Don't get me wrong, making it through the collegiate and medical education process takes a high level of confidence. It is an accomplishment that should be respected. That being said, there are individuals that come through the system with a sense of self that prompts behaviors which impact trust and relationships.

## THE PROVIDER AS A PROFESSIONAL

"The Patient may be safer with a physician who is naturally wise than one who is artificially learned"
Theordore Fox

The healthcare provider plays a number of direct and indirect roles within the healthcare environment including managing and caring for their patient and patient's families, being leaders in addressing quality of care, and teaching and mentoring other healthcare providers. They are leaders in public health, responsible for contributing to a sustainable healthcare system and often have fiduciary and leadership roles in healthcare organizations including hospitals, health systems, healthcare services organizations and insurance companies. These roles are all complex and sometimes appear to be in conflict with each other. What is common across all of these roles is the importance of trust.

The Robert Wood Johnson Foundation and the National Institute on Health looked at the issue of trust, honesty and integrity of physicians as healers, as well as healthcare leaders. The research looked at the years 1966 to 2014. In 1966, 75% of Americans had confidence in providers and healthcare. Unfortunately, this level dropped to 34% by 2012. Interestingly across this same timeframe, physician's integrity remains high at 69%. Those surveyed stated that physicians were honest and ethical as a group. The question is why is there conflicting sentiment in the data? A great deal of it may be attributed to societal trust as a whole. Physicians are often swept into the trust tsunami. Only 23 % of the public surveyed stated that they had confidence in the system (Gallup 2014). It may also be that the decreased trust is not due to things such as honesty and integrity but changes in expectations and relationships.

Clearly, healthcare providers, especially physicians go through many years of competitive education. At the end of their training many providers place themselves on a pedestal of sorts. This can create situations where providers often have problems judging their own performance with consumers. The GE Camden 2016 study found that 63% of providers believed that they were delivering a good health experience while consumers felt that the care delivered was good only 40% of the time. A further breakdown of the experience found

"Provider take the time to understand my needs and explain options"
| | |
|---|---|
| Providers | 51% believed that this was the case |
| Consumers | 34% believed that this was the case |

"Providers have empathy"
| | |
|---|---|
| Providers | 57% believed that this was the case |
| Consumers | 36% believed that this was the case. |

GE Camden

Changes in trust within healthcare, whatever the reason have not gone unnoticed. In 2018, The American Board of Internal Medicine began an initiative that looked at the intersection of the provider and their impact on trust. The initiative focused on how trust impacts healthcare outcomes, patient satisfaction and physician well-being. Along with research, the foundation has created the" Trust Challenge." The challenge identifies examples of where incorporating trust in the healthcare experience has had a positive influence on these three outcomes. Their goal is to share these actions across providers and enhance the experience to create a strong and trusting relationship between the provider and those that they serve.

The changes that have occurred in healthcare including payment models, organizational models and relationships have made an impact on the American healthcare provider. There is an increasing concern about provider burnout. In this case, burnout includes emotional and physical exhaustion. A 2018 study by Medscape found that 42% of the 15,000 providers that they surveyed have been impacted by burnout. We know that provider engagement is an important factor for trust. Although there is not a single agreed upon definition for provider engagement, we do know that engagement includes "those who are involved in, enthusiastic about and committed to their work." Engagement requires an emotional commitment. Patients sense when their doctor is engaged. (Kruse, Forbes) Unfortunately, provider burnout challenges their ability to connect with peers and patients. In addition, the lack of energy reduces their ability to feel engaged and empathic. Lack of empathy leads to the destruction of the relationship and reduction of trust.

In 2017, in response to the increasing concerns regarding physician burnout the AMA made changes to their Code of Ethics. Prior to this period both the AMA Code of Ethics and the Hippocratic oath focused on the responsibility of the provider to the patient by placing the welfare of the patient above all else including the physician themselves. The changes to the Code of Ethics spoke of placing a greater focus on physician self -care with the hope that this would reduce burnout. When we interviewed patients and asked them about this, several admitted to mixed feelings. Most did agree that physicians should take care of themselves. Others stated that physicians should be taking care of themselves on "their own time" and that physicians were being paid to take care of them as a patient. A couple stated that physicians have been taking care of themselves for years by limiting hours of care and not being available in the evening and weekends.

At the end of the day, trust makes work more enjoyable for providers. It is not gratifying to work all day with those that you do not trust. One provider described it as being on a battlefield with each man and woman protecting themselves.

## Provider and Communication

### Words Matter

How we communicate goes a long way to creating a trusting relationship. Communication can be used for information giving, information gathering, information verifying, an emotional interaction or a way to show interest and respect. Regardless of the purpose, if communication is done poorly there will be a significant impact on trust regardless who is involved.

Like countries having their own language, many professions, including healthcare providers, have their own lingo. Healthcare executives also have their own "language." As healthcare providers experience the training process, they begin to learn a new vocabulary, medical jargon. A rite of passage. It happens slowly but consistently throughout the educational process. Many of us are unaware of this change. The words and language that we speak as healthcare professional often communicate our knowledge to other healthcare providers. It is a way to show that you belong to a "club." Medical jargon has been found to be a two -edged sword. On the one hand, it has been shown to create trust from the listener. Dr. Joe is more trustworthy because he is really smart and fluent in the knowledge of medicine. This contrasts with medical jargon being used and the receiver not understanding and feeling like they are being belittled or disrespected. The jargon has created a barrier to those that do not understand the words.

Over the last few years understanding of the importance of communication in healthcare has increased. A growing number of medical schools have formal communication skills programs. In talking to healthcare providers, we have heard differing opinions regarding the focus on communications.

> Georgia is a 45- year-old physician. When asked about her beliefs on communication and trust, Georgia shared "I find it kind of funny, we spend time learning new terms and how to practice medicine and now we need to spend time unlearning what we learned." I must admit, the retraining that I got on health literacy probably helped me. I did not even realize the amount of medical terminology I was using. I probably sounded like a medical nerd. I think that my patients appreciate that I am talking with them in a way that they can understand. I wonder how many of my patients were shaking their heads while I spoke and did not understand what I was saying to them"

In addition to medical jargon, communication habits and styles can create or destroy trust. Each of us have habits that are attached to our communication style. Are we more verbose? Do we go into greater detail or are we more succinct? Are we more formal or more personal in our style? Howard Beckman and Richard Frankel published a study in 1984 that addresses a common communication challenge for providers, "the interruption." Their study found that on average a physician interrupts a patient's after 18 seconds of speaking. This study has been replicated a number of times over the years with similar outcomes. There are a number of reasons that these interruptions occur. In some cases, providers are concerned that the patient will "just keep on talking" and this will put the provider behind in their daily schedule. Other reasons include the desire to maintain control in the patient/doctor relationship. Most providers do not understand that interrupting the patient may be perceived as rude or disrespectful. Interestingly, there are some occasions where the provider interrupting the patient can help to focus a patient. If this is the case, sharing this information as to why they are interrupting can help maintain the respect that is an important ingredient to trust.

> Julies, a middle-aged schoolteacher shared that he was meeting with his doctor for an annual visit. He had prepared for the visit by writing down those things that he wanted to talk to his doctor about. During the conversation he went from discussing issues he had with indigestion and then began sharing issues with insomnia. He shared that his doctor interrupted him as he changed topics. At first this upset Jules until his doctor actually stated, "I am sorry that I am interrupting you, but I would like to stay on the subject of your indigestion prior to going on to your next issue. This will help me to better understand the issue." Jules went from being frustrated with his doctor to appreciating that his doctor was both actually listening to him and that he cared.

Incongruency in our unspoken and spoken messaging is the third common communication factor that can often create challenges to the trust relationship. Most of us do not realize that 93% of what we communicate is based on our non-verbal communication.

> Dr Jonas is a 61- year- old Internal Medicine provider as well as the Chief Medical Officer of a hospital system. He shared an experience that created a moment of "embarrassing self-awareness." "The last thing I do with each patient is to ask them if they have any additional questions. One of my patients got very mad at me and pointed out that he was asking this as he was walking out the door of the exam room. The patient

went on to tell me that he felt I was being rude and dismissive. I apologized but silently felt that the patient was oversensitive. Two days later, I was speaking with the President of the hospital that I am an administrator at. As we were finishing up a business conversation, he asked me if I had any further thoughts. His hand was on the conference room doorknob. Suddenly, I understood my patient's response to my incongruency of action, my asking a question but not really wanting him to answer it."

Communication incongruency is not the only communication skill that Dr Jonas had to address. He shared his having to learn how to better communicate with his healthcare executive colleagues. Dr Jonas learned that how he communicates with his patients and fellow providers was different than how he has communicated with his healthcare executive peers.

The first six months as a Chief Medical Officer at the hospital was a real learning experience. Hospital administrators use different terms and speak in a different cadence. I had to learn that in order to be respected and trusted, I had to use business terms and shorten up my conversation.

Dr Jonas was not the only one that had to learn that lesson. This is a lesson that I too had to learn. As the Chief Medical Officer of a Fortune 100 company, I reported to the CEO of the company. He was known to have a short attention span. I had to learn to give my opinion or ask my questions in less than 30 seconds. This required me to practice at home with a timer. I have passed this advice to many of my provider colleagues that are transitioning to business roles. I found that I had to consciously "code switch" depending on whether I was speaking with a consumer, a provider, peer or fellow healthcare executive. This variation in linguistic norm is now something that I can do seamlessly and without conscious effort. It has become a skill that has become invaluable in creating a trusting relationship with each of these stakeholders.

## Provider and Consumer

> "Physicians are intellectually and morally
> obligated advocates for their patients."
> Hippocrates

The relationship between the physician and the patient is founded in trust. We have talked about the trust of the consumer to the provider. We need to remember that trust the is not uni-directional. When studied, it has become increasingly apparent that there is a reduction of trust from the provider to the consumer as well. Historically, doctors have believed that their patients trusted them because that is what they were supposed to do. It was expected. To a large extent, this was true in the past. Unfortunately, this is no longer the case.

The role of the provider as a trusted teacher and healer has existed for centuries. Trust has been a foundational attribute assigned to providers as they delivered on these roles. As healthcare has evolved, the relationship between a doctor and a patient has changed. These changes require different types of relationships and different motivators or detractors of trust. The previous relationship was based on a paternal model, Robert Truog described it as "benevolent paternalism." Over the last several years there has been a shift in the relationship away from the paternalistic model to one of more equality where respect and empathy are dominant activities. Robert Truog speaks of the evolution of the patient and physician relationship. The question is has this change in relationship created a change in trust? (Truog, 2012)

Dr. Jain is a pediatrician. She lives in the same community as many of her patients. In order to prepare for her workday, Dr. Jay reviews her patient list. This does two things, it allows her to take care of any preparation work she needs prior to seeing a patient, it also allows her to review any personal attributes or nuances about each of the patient's that she will be seeing. This is something that she learned from one of her mentors. "By having these personal conversations with my patients, it is easier for them to trust me when I have something distressing to tell them"

You will often hear the phrase, "nothing about me, without me." In order to achieve this consumer desired goal, the relationship has had to evolve towards a more equal type of partnership. In order for this to work both parties need to both listen and trust each other. It is a division of expertise, power and labor.

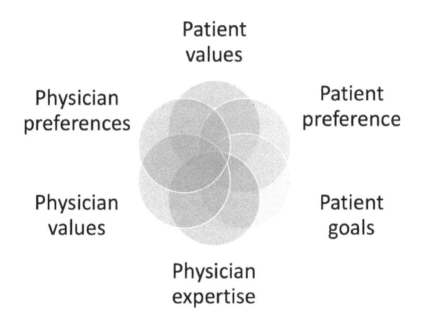

**Source: Health Intelligence Partners**

This evolution in roles has created different expectations. Unfortunately, the expectations and goals of the relationship are rarely aligned. This lack of alignment can create dis-satisfaction and increased levels of mistrust. In fact, there are a number of signs that the trust that has long been linked to providers is at now at risk. A 2016 Gallup poll found that American physicians did not fair particularly well when consumers were asked the question "All things considered, doctors in the U.S. can be trusted." The United States ranked 24th in the answer to this question. (Lynch T, Wolfson D. Baron R. A Trust Initiative in Healthcare: Why and Why Now? Academic Medicine. 94(4) April 2019 pp. 463-465).

How do providers, especially physicians feel about this ranking? Not surprisingly, the provider response is not uniform.

> Dr. Delbert is a 55-year-old ophthalmologist. He has led a six-person practice for over 25 years. When asked whether he felt his patients trusted him, Dilbert replied "of course my patients trust me, I studied for years at top universities, I trained at top hospitals and I have never been sued. Why wouldn't they trust me? Besides, if they did not trust me, I am sure that they would not continue to see me."

> Dr. Carl is a 51-year-old pediatrician. He works as part of a large multi-specialty practice. We asked Carl, a similar question about whether he believes that his patients and their families trust him. "Wow, I hope so. I know that clinically I stay up to date. In addition, I have spent years getting to know these families. I would be really disappointed if they did not trust me. If that is the case. I have failed as a doctor.

"Medicine is a moral enterprise grounded in the covenant of trust." Crawshaw in his paper stated that "physicians are morally obligated to act as advocates for the sick wherever their welfare is threatened and for their health at all times" (Crawshaw et al, 1995). The Physician/Patient Covenant as published in JAMA states that health professionals have three obligations associated with being trustworthy; they have to have high levels of judgment and skill known as competence, second, they must act consistently for the good of the patient, and third they need to fulfill special role such as fiduciary roles. Dr. Delbert's response focuses the competence form of trust. The historical belief of "assumed trust" has been primarily associated with education and expertise still exists in many people like Dr. Dilbert. As you can see from Dr. Carl, an increasing number of providers are beginning to understand that competence is not the only factor that plays into gaining and maintaining trust with their patients. In Carl's case, trust is also focused on the relationship he has with his patients and their families. (JAMA). Although they agree that trust is important, they understand the concept in different ways.

The AMA Physician/Patient Covenant also speaks about the fiduciary relationship between the two stakeholders. If you go back to a time prior to health insurance as we know it today, the financial relationship was totally between the physician and the patient. The patient came to the physician for care and then paid them for their services. The cost of care was transparent, and the patient paid the physician directly. Over the last 40 years, this model has transformed. The question is whether this change has created a change in the fiduciary role of the provider and whether this fiduciary change has impacted trust.

In addition to direct trust, (between a healthcare provider and their patient), indirect trust also exists through the transfer of trust. The transfer of trust by a primary care provider to another healthcare professional is an integral part of healthcare. This is true regardless of whether the consumer has had a previous relationship with this other provider or not. It does not matter if the new provider is within the same office of the primary care provider, through a referral to a specialist or to a hospital. As we have discussed, healthcare is a team event, and it is common for there to be multiple providers involved in the consumer's care. The role of the primary care provider transferring trust between themselves and their patients (family and caregivers included in this) to other members within the healthcare environment has become increasingly important in the era of patient centered medical homes, ACOs and other new organizational models in which a more team-oriented approach is common.

> George is a 52-year-old male. He had been quite healthy most of his life. Recently on a visit to his primary care physician, he was diagnosed with an inguinal hernia that although was benign, due to its size needed to be removed. George did not have a surgeon, so he asked his primary care doctor for a referral. He trusted his doctor and felt that this was the best way to receive high level quality care. On his first visit to the surgeon, George found the doctor to be a bit brusque but chose to stay with the surgeon because he felt his primary care doctor would not mislead him.

We often speak about the importance of a consumer trusting their healthcare providers. The topic of providers trusting their patients does not often arise. Why is that? Is providers trust in the consumer as important as consumer trust in their providers? Is it assumed that this trust exists? What causes providers to distrust their patients? These are areas that have been less researched. Linda Girgis in her blog stated that there is no stronger bond than between a doctor and patient with the exception of marriage. It is a matter of life and death. (Girgis, 2018). Honest and open conversations are the cornerstone of a good provider/patient relationship Doctors need to trust their patients so that they can get the information that they need to support the consumer in their health and healthcare needs. Research has found that when a doctor does not trust their patient, their patients tend not to trust them. "Failure to listen to patients is often the first manifestation of inadequate trust" (Grob R, Darien G, Meyers D. Why physicians should trust in patients. JAMA. 2019; 321(14) pp 1347-1348)

Geona shares that there was a 10- year period when she would not tell her doctor that she was a lesbian. She was not sure if the doctor would "fire her, judge her or treat her differently." I did not know the doctor well, did not know their politics or how they felt about the gay and lesbian community. Because of that, I just stayed silent. I did not lie but I did not disclose. Kind of a don't ask, don't tell posture."

Providers concern over patients withholding information or lying to them is not unfounded. A TermLife2Go 2020 survey asked 500 Americans a number of questions about their conversations with their doctors. The survey found that 23%, almost one in four consumers lie to their doctor at some point throughout their relationship. The lies vary from, 46% stating that they lie about their smoking habits, while just short of that at 43% lie about how much exercise they participate in. 38% were not truthful about their how much alcohol they consume. 29% did not tell the truth about their sexual partners. When asked as to why they had withheld the truth or had lied, their reasons were similar to those articulated by Georgia.

- 31% said that they lied to avoid discrimination
- 22% lied because that did not think that their doctor would take them seriously
- Many stated that they told the provider what they believed the provider wanted to hear.
- Many were concerned that their provider would judge them, be mad at them, yell at them or "fire them"
- One lied because he did not want to be lectured by his doctor
- One lied because a parent was in the room and they did not want to share their sexual activity in from of their parent
                              (TermLife2Go.com.February 24, 2020)

Lifestyle activities are not the only areas in which individuals withhold information or lie to their provider. Trust between a provider and consumer has been shown to have a significant impact on the consumers adherence to care. How do healthcare providers feel their patients withholding information about being non-adherent? Providers, like all individuals, get angry and frustrated when they find that their patients are not following the care that they advise or prescribe. In addition to not following instructions, providers are furthered frustrated by the fact that their patients often are not honest about their lack of adherence. This emotional response can begin a cascade of distrust between the patient and the doctor. It may also impact not only distrust in the specific patient but patients in general.

Providers, like all people, do not like to have people withhold the truth. For healthcare providers the stakes are often higher than between two individuals in other areas of business or personally. Individuals such as Dr. Delbert, admit to not understand why their patients do not follow their recommendations.

> "As I shared with you, I have spent a great deal of time getting educated in my specialty, the patient has not. Do they think that they know more than I do? It frustrates me and makes me mad. I don't know why they just don't listen. If they have questions or a problem with what I am telling them, they need to tell me. Otherwise, they are wasting my time."

Other providers we spoke to were more concerned about the potential impact of non- adherence.

> Dr Patel is a 47-year-old physician that spoke about his thoughts around non- adherence to his treatment plans. "My test and treatment plans are based on the best scientific knowledge and guidelines that exist. In addition, I have discussed this with my patient. The tests, procedures and prescriptions that I recommend will help the patient to have the best outcomes possible. I hate to think that the

patient would not follow my directions and then get worse, or even die. No doctor wants that. We go into medicine to help people."

Dr Belgium, a 50-year-old pediatrician talks about her patients and their parents that refuse to receive their vaccinations. "I gave them the science behind the vaccines as well as the risks and benefits of the vaccine. We spent a great deal of time discussing this. Unfortunately, they continued to refuse all vaccines for their children. They state that they trust me and that they just have a different view of vaccines. There has been a great deal of talk about what to do in this case. I documented the discussions well in the chart. I decided not to "fire" the family from my practice. I am hoping that over time that they will change their mind"

One area that Dr Patel, Dr Belgium and Dr Delbert agree upon is that lying and withholding important information, creates a distrust that can significantly degrade the relationship between the individuals. At the very least, it creates a skeptic of the person that was lied to. It is not unusual for someone that has been lied to, to question things that the other individual says in the future. In other cases, the trust bond has been broken and the individual lied to trusts little or nothing that the other person says. We asked each of the providers we spoke to regarding lying and/or non-adherence about actions that they take. Their responses varied from those similar to Dr. Belgium that documented the interactions to those that dismiss the patient and/or family from the practice. These responses are similar to the work of Dr Schroeder in his work with 30 providers. This group was asked to list the reasons why they fired patients from their practice. Although the main reason was the patient abusing either the doctor or the medical staff, interestingly compliance, physician intuition and trust were also found on the list. (Schroeder, CA, Why Physicians Fire Patients: My Informal

Survey, Patient Care Consultant Live, January 3, 2019). Whether providers only documented the lies once revealed, documented the non-adherence to advice or dismissed the consumer from their practice, all of the providers discussed their concerns over potential malpractice concerns.

# Evolving Relationship

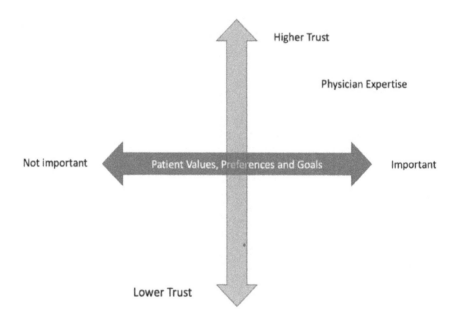

**Source: Health Intelligence Partners**

The providers that we spoke to, whether they were more like Delbert or Carl, all shared their frustration with how their relationship with their patient is changing. Most talked about going into medicine to help people. A significant number spoke of their family's experiences with physicians and how they wanted to either emulate these past experiences or to create better experiences for their patients than their family had. Many primary care providers spoke about their desire for long term relationships with their patients and their families. For many, there was almost a sadness in their tone as they spoke about the diminishing of trust

## Provider and Provider

As science has advanced and healthcare has become more complex, the historic model of one patient: one provider is diminishing. Healthcare is no longer the dyad it once was. It is an intertwined set of interactions between professionals, somewhat similar to a team sport. Like a team sport, all the players have to coordinate and trust one another.

Richard Frankle and his colleagues discuss that providers are not only challenged in trusting their patients, but they also often have difficulties trusting each other. The lack of trust between providers is caused by some of the same reasons as consumers and providers not trusting each other. Historically, healthcare providers knew each other; their children went to school together and they often prayed together. The referral patterns between providers were based on these personal relationships. This is no longer the case. Today, referral networks are created by the Health Insurance Plans or the Health Systems that providers work for or contract with. It is not unusual for these networks to change regularly. This fluidity can be a challenge in building strong lasting relationships. This challenge has also created a culture of mistrust between physicians. (Frankel RM, Tilden VP et al)

Physicians deal with non-physician colleagues as well. The healthcare provider community is made up of a large, varied group of professionals which include nurses, physician assistants, pharmacists, mental health providers, nutritionists and many others. All of these individuals make up the healthcare team. All need to trust each other in order to achieve the desired goal of efficient and effective healthcare.

In order to understand the challenges in trust between healthcare professionals one needs to appreciate some of the dynamics. The 2018

American Board of Internal Medicine Foundation Forum on trust focused on some of the barriers to trust. They included areas such as how to co-manage patients across providers, issues of mutual respect and communication and other behaviors that can impact trust.

> Dr Johal is a cardiologist in a mid-size midwestern city. Dr. Johal shared his thoughts about working with and trusting other providers. "Most of my patients have complicated heart disease along with a number of other medical problems.There are usually at least 3 or 4 other doctors that are treating my patients. When asked if he trusted these other providers he shared, "in most cases, I do not know who these other individuals are. I did not choose them for my patients and I rarely speak with them. Do I trust them, on the one hand, I have to assume that they are appropriately trained but on the other hand, I don't know them? Hard to trust someone you don't know"

It is not unusual for individuals to be co-managed by several providers. Most providers focus on their area of expertise. As Johal shared, communication between these providers is rare. This can create a situation where one provider may contradict another physician's decision. In some cases, this occurs unknowingly, in other cases, such as with second opinions, it may be that there is a disagreement in what care is appropriate. As Paracelsus stated, medicine is not only a science; it is also an art. There is not always one right answer. In order for co-management to occur in a trustful and appropriate manner for all involved it is important that communication and respect come into play. Only most recently, has there been increased conversation about providers interacting more for the benefit of the patient.

In 1996, the role of the hospitalist began to be formalized. These physicians, nurse practitioners and physician assistant's role are to care for individuals during their hospital stays. The hospitalist model makes a great deal of sense as it allows for a group of professionals to focus all their time and energy on those that are in acute need.

Historically, healthcare professionals had to juggle their ambulatory patients with those that were in the hospital. This was not always easy. Unfortunately, communication is rare between the hospitalist and the ambulatory care team of a patient. This can create a number of unfortunate situations, such as providers second guessing each other or in some cases disparaging each other. Not only can this lead to mistrust between the healthcare professionals it can also lead to trust issues with the patient.

> Dr. Deborah is a 61-year-old pediatrician. Deborah shared that it is not just the negative dynamic between the hospitalist and the ambulatory providers that affects communication and respect. "this is not a new issue. I trained in the early 1980s. Even back then, there was distrust between the academic doctors and the community doctors. As residents we saw this all the time. Our attendings during training were always criticizing the community doctors. It was almost like a competition. Unfortunately, this behavior became a learned behavior as one left residency"

As in many professions, hierarchies and power dynamics in healthcare exist. Most often we think of these occurring between different types of healthcare providers. In other cases, they occur within one type of provider group.

> Let's return to Dr. Deborah. After finishing her pediatric residency, Deborah joined a 12- provider general pediatric group. Today she leads this group. Deborah shares that the group consists of pediatricians, pediatric nurse practitioners, a social worker, a pharmacist and a pediatric nutritionist. "We each have our roles. We were trained to know different things. I could not do their

jobs and they could not do my job. This is not only good for our patients. It is great for me. I learn something new every day. We trust each other with our patient's lives."

This trust across different healthcare providers is not always the case. The reasons for the lack of trust are multifaceted. In some cases, it is due to economic competitiveness. This has been the case between nurse practitioners and physicians for many years. Some say that the competition is not due to financial competition but "a training and knowledge difference." In a 2019 Medical Economics article, Todd Shryock spoke about how some physicians did not trust that nurse practitioners were trained in a way that would allow them to practice independently. They spoke about the issue in terms of patient safety.

Trust challenges do not just occur between nurse practitioners and doctors. Over the last 20 years we have seen this type of trust challenge increase between pharmacists and physicians. As medications have taken on a greater role in both healthcare and healthcare economics, the interactions between pharmacists and prescribing providers (physicians, nurse practitioners, and physician assistants, etc.). It is not unusual for a pharmacist to reach out to a prescribing provider to suggest a change in prescription due to either a safety issue or a situation where a consumer can save money through a generic or comparable medicine. This information is not always accepted in a professional manner.

Let's return to Dr Delbert, the ophthalmologist that we spoke about earlier. We discussed medication management with him. "My office gets 100s of calls from pharmacies and the drug management companies telling us we should change our patient's prescriptions. They may know medicines, but they don't know our patients. They should trust us. We know what we are doing"

I want to take a moment and speak a bit more about pharmacists. In 1998, I joined a pharmacy benefit management organization. During my medical education and then early in my medical career, I learned to understand the importance of my healthcare provider colleagues. I, like Dr Deborah could not imagine practicing medicine without these professional individuals. The one area that I had limited interaction with was pharmacists. Although I had worked in a neighborhood pharmacy as a teenager, I really had little understanding of the education and knowledge that pharmacists possess. I know that they dispensed medicines that I prescribed. It was not until joining Caremark that I began to understand and respect the profession. Today, I rarely will prescribe or take a medication without seeking input from a pharmacist colleague. I trust them more than I trust myself regarding medication management.

It is not just between different provider types where hierarchy and trust issues exist. It also occurs within provider types. As the number of medical specialties have increased over the last fifty years, so has the hierarchal nature of the medical profession. Interactions based on power and not on relationships or trust have developed. The assumption of trust due to mutual education and status as a physician breaks down when we look at the relationship and trust within the medical community. Doctors are competitive. This competitiveness comes from years of education where an individual is competing with another for grades, places in medical school and residency positions. It also comes from the environment in which they exist. Dr. Deborah shared with us the competition, lack of respect and lack of trust between academic physicians and community- based physicians. This also occurs across medical specialties. It is not unusual for a physician with a specialty to feel superior to those in primary care. The lack of respect between specialties is another cause of distrust between providers. Academic providers are often known to state that community providers are "not real doctors." This is not new as we often heard our academic attendings say this about the local community physicians as far back as they 1980s. It is also not unusual to hear a specialist state that the patient's primary care provider made a bad decision because they have "limited training. (Frankel et al. 2019).

Regardless of the reason, it is common for there to be trust fractures between healthcare providers as well as across the healthcare stakeholder environment. Whether due to competitive reasons or lack of understanding of the expertise that each provider brings to the table, trust fractures such these negatively impact the healthcare system.

There is one aspect of trust betweeen healthcare providers that few speak about. It is much more enjoyable to work with those that you respect and trust. The energy that it takes to work in a dysfunctional, non-trusting or toxic environment is significant. As we often spend more time with our co-workers than our families, it is important that these are people that bring energy to our lives and not extract energy out.

## Providers and Healthcare Executives

> Dr Saala is an Internal Medicine physician that has been in practice for 15 years. He shared with us his feelings about his interactions with different healthcare executives. "They clearly do not respect me as an equal. The underlying message in our conversations is that I should stick to treating patients."

The Hippocratic oath and medical ethics organizations have stated that physicians should be exclusively focused on the best interest of the patient. Norman Levinsky "physicians are required to do everything that they believe may benefit each patient without regard to costs or other societal consideration" (Levinsky NG. NEJM). The challenge to these beliefs is that the delineation between care and costs are not always clear cut. This has become increasingly true over the last 40 years as healthcare has in some ways become more corporate in nature. Clinicians have become more circumspect and leerier of the motives of the healthcare system and the world in which they work. The social movement of the 1960s encouraged "distrust." I remember the adage of "never trust anyone over 30" We questioned everything during that time period. Authority of any type was the "bad guy."

Doctors were not immune to that mindset. For a period of time, this distrust of authority was reduced. Unfortunately, the changing healthcare environment such as the advent of HMOs in the 1990's brought this level of distrust back to the surface. As healthcare continues to change and creates new models of care and payment distrust continues to exist.

Mark Hertling, a retired Lt. General of the U.S. Army has written a book titled, "Growing Physician Leaders." In the book he states that lack of trust between physicians and healthcare administrators is the greatest challenge facing the two groups. Hertling and others have found several reasons that trust is hard to attain between these two groups: including lack of respect, communication challenges and misalignment of goals. A 2019 article in JAMA by Louis Sandy, outlined and articulated a trust model between providers and healthcare executives that included competence, transparency and motive as his three foundational areas of trust. You will note that Hertling and Sandy's models are closely aligned.

Jim Collins in his book, *Good to Great* talks about the importance of both respect and trust in creating great working relationships and teams. In order to have respect, one has to understand the knowledge and value that an individual brings to the partnership. It is not unusual for physicians to be pigeon- holed as clinicians or "Ivory Tower executives" and therefore not able to understand business. It is perceived that a provider's competence is focused on clinical care. In return, physicians often perceive that the lack of medical education by many healthcare executives creates a void in the executives caring about the patient. The provider cannot conceive that a healthcare executive is unable to understand compassion and desire for a positive outcome for the consumer. This often creates frustration and the fracture of trust between providers and healthcare executives.

Like respect, communication discordance often creates barriers to trust. Providers and healthcare executives both utilize the words, jargon and concepts that are familiar to their roles. These two languages often create misunderstanding and can end in a communication standoff. Are these communication differences unconscious or are they being used as weapons?

Over the last 10 years, the creation of a trusting relationship between healthcare providers and executives has become even more acute and important as their professional relationships have evolved. Over the last several years healthcare has integrated vertically whereas hospitals, healthcare systems and insurance companies have begun to acquire and employ healthcare providers. Unfortunately, these relationships are often based on business and not on trust. Providers also often do not trust these large organizations that they currently report to. You may ask; why are healthcare providers choosing to become employed by organizations that they do not trust? The answers vary and are not simple. Often, the groups feel that they do not have a choice in this increasingly complex healthcare environment. In other cases, the providers looked to large organizations in order to take care of the business aspects of their healthcare practices. This allowed them to concentrate on what they loved most and studied for years to do; take care of patients. The issue became that they then felt that they lost some control on the practice of medicine. In addition, it is often the first time the provider is reporting into a non-clinical staff member. Providers, like other individuals, do not automatically trust those that may think differently from them. This lack of concurrence or blind trust takes time to overcome. The lack of trust in these situations is based on  factors that we have already touched upon; lack of understanding and perceived misalignment of goals.

Dr Quint is a physician that for many years practiced medicine within a practice with 7 other clinicians. Three years ago, the group sold their practice to a large health system that also acted as a health insurance company. When Dr Quint and the group were told that they needed to change how they communicated with their patients, he became angry. "Clearly, they do not understand how our practice works "This anger then created a trust chasm that bled into other organizational interactions. This lack of trust and at times outright anger, took three years to overcome. "I am not sure that I totally trust them today. Now it is more like, trust but confirm, working relationship"

It will be interesting to see if these issues of trust change as young healthcare providers join corporate practices earlier in their careers. As this occurs, there is some level of optimism. When you speak with healthcare providers that began their careers in a corporate healthcare structure such as Kaiser Permanente, there seems to be a higher degree of trust.

I spoke to Mary Felipe, a nurse practitioner and her husband Chris, an internal medicine doctor. They both talked about joining a Kaiser practice right out of training. Dr Felipe shared that his peers often ask him if he feels that he is limited in what he does. "We love what we do and where we do it. We believe that we can practice good medicine. We want the same thing that the company wants, quality healthcare. So far there is no reason to not trust them."

## Provider and Hospital/Health Systems

A doctor is judged only by his patients and immediate colleagues, that is, behind closed doors, man to man"
Milan Kundera, author, The Unbearable Lightness of Being

Doctors have had a long relationship with hospitals. The relationship was based on an established interdependency. This is where doctors admitted their patients to receive care for serious acute conditions.

They needed to trust the hospital to offer the care that these patients required. Although the hospital offered the real estate and the tools, the providers controlled what and how care was given. The decision making and power structure of the hospital during this time was focused on the medical staff organization. This group of individuals (mostly physicians) had a great deal of influence on the hospital administrators and therefore the decision- making processes of the hospital. Over the last thirty years, the provider/hospital relationship has changed.

In 1992, Paul Starr talked about the changing relationship between physicians and hospitals due to the reduction in the healthcare providers "autonomy, authority and ability to self -regulate." (Starr P. *The Social Transformation of American Medicine*. Basic Books 1982.). Provider oversight activities such as utilization management (UM) began to appear. Utilization management created a "mother may I" type of relationship between the provider and the hospital. Although these activities began in the 1960's, significant oversight did not occur until the late 1980s. By 1992, the review of services requested by providers for their patients became ubiquitous. In addition, diagnosis-related groups, DRGs, began to be used in the 1980s. The combination of UM and DRGs were significant drivers in the change in relationship and reduction of trust between healthcare organizations and providers. The financial arrangements between hospital systems and doctors have created a further perception of loss of autonomy for the provider. They feel these organizations look out for their own best interest not that of the doctor or the patient. The provider feels that they know what is best for their patient. This creates a sense of misaligned goals and degradation of trust.

In addition to changes in power and autonomy between hospitals and providers, providers have difficulties trusting hospitals due their institutional makeup. It is hard to trust inanimate objects. There is no "who to trust." It used to be if there was a disagreement, a provider would talk with the medical staff organization in order to get support. It is perceived that this group no longer has significant influence with the leadership of the hospital. Historically, many hospitals were led by physicians. Today, 5% of hospitals have physicians as CEO. This number has decreased by 90% since 1935. There has been a great deal of discussion regarding this trend. It is often stated that physicians are very good at treating patients but do not have the knowledge and expertise to run a hospital system.

> Nigel is the CEO of a 10- hospital system. Nigel talked about his interactions with the providers that work within and admit patients to his hospital. "They are practitioners and not businesspeople" "would you trust your car mechanic to act as your financial advisor." During our conversation I shared with Nigel that out of the 21 hospitals added to the 2029 U.S. News and World Report "Best Hospitals" list more than half had physician CEO. (Gupta, 2019). Nigel had no response to this statistic. Nigel went on to say "The doctors that I know well, I like. I golf with them. my wife and I have dinner with them. I trust them as good humans. I just don't necessarily trust them to help run a hospital"

## Provider and Health Plans

Trust takes a lifetime to build, seconds to break and forever to repair
Dhar Mann

One of the most contentious, least trusting relationships within healthcare over the last 30 years is between the healthcare provider and the health plans. In 1982, Paul Starr predicted that this issue would begin to challenge the healthcare industry. One of the reasons for this decrease in trust was that physicians felt their autonomy and decision-making capability was being reduced by healthcare organizations. This discomfort, frustration and even anger has persisted and in fact increased over the last 30 years. The relationship between providers and health plans has been compared to David and Goliath; between those that care for the patient and the large organizations that pay for much of the care. In many ways, Starr's prediction has come true.

The Physician/Patient Covenant as discussed earlier, not only speaks about competence but also of the duty of the provider to assure care in the best interest of the patient. Over the last 25 years, healthcare providers frequently articulated frustration and concern that health plans are a barrier to this obligation. This frustration leads to a fracturing of trust between the two stakeholders.

> Dr. Lyle is a physician that is employed by a large organization. Sometimes he experiences conflict feeling he is "reporting" to two masters. There are some areas that have conflicting priorities which interferes with success. Sometimes he wants to order tests to make the patient feel more comfortable with his diagnosis but knows that society and his employer want him to be more cost conscious. In the end, he feels overall that he acts on behalf of his patients, that is why he became a doctor, but it is hard. He believes that the trust covenant is being tested and threatened in today's environment.

This breakdown of trust is the product of a number of issues between the provider and the Health Plan including power, misaligned goals, financial issues, administrative inefficiencies and perceived quality issues. Over the last 30 years, Health Plans, like hospitals, have been able to approve or disapprove care decisions that are made between the provider and their patient. This model of utilization management has a bifurcated purpose of both cost and quality. The Dartmouth Atlas project which began in 1993, found significant variation of care across the United States. It was perceived by Health Plans that this variation had an impact on both the costs and quality of healthcare being delivered by providers. The Dartmouth Atlas along with rising healthcare costs, created the utilization management model that still exists today. The 11th Annual Revive Trust Index found that physicians discovered significant hassles and barriers to giving care to their patients from the health plans due to UM programs. They felt that the payment models were not aligned and put the patient and the provider at a disadvantage. Providers feel that UM creates a system where the Health Plan is playing too great a role in the care of the patient. They see this as intrusive and inappropriate. There have been attempts by the health plans to mute these feelings using provider committees that create and oversee the UM programs that exist within the health plan. In some cases, these types of committees have been able to reduce the lack of trust between the two groups but for the most part, UM programs are still seen as a barrier to trust

> Dr Sally is a primary care physician that also acts as the Chief Medical Officer of a Health Plan. One of Dr Sally's roles is to oversee the utilization management program offered to the Health Plans' clients. When talking to Dr Sally about the issues associated with trust between her, the other healthcare providers and the Health Plan, she shared the following story, "I was very excited to take on the role of Chief Medical Officer. I felt that I could bring value to both the patients within the plan, my fellow doctors and the Health Plan itself. What I found out was that behind my back I was called a traitor by my peers and not trusted by the plan to act in the plans best interest. It really sucked to not be trusted by anyone."

Over the last few years, the two stakeholders have begun to enter in new types of contractual arrangements. The 2010 Affordable Care Act put into motion contractual arrangements that replaced fee for volume with fee for value. The purpose of these new contractual models is to create better alignment of incentives and hopefully to increase trust. As we know trust does not appear overnight. The Revive 2017 survey found that only 55.8% of physicians trust health plans. This is during a time that the Plans believe that there is significantly improved relationship. The providers still believe that the plans are not "fair" to them or their patients and that they are the only stakeholder that has the knowledge to act in the patient's best interest. The fractured relationship and lack of trust of providers to the health plans was discussed at the 2018 American Board of Internal Medicine Forum on Trust. Providers at the forum did agree that Health Plans do bring value through the execution of their core business activities including paying claims, aggregating data and communicating healthcare policy. In addition, they understand that these things can positively impact both the provider and the consumer improving the trust between themselves and the health plan. Old feelings die hard. It will take time to see if the two stakeholders begin to build trust. Hopefully, that trust will increase as older providers retire and younger providers who never transitioned from independent decision making to one that has oversight by the health plan increasingly take their place. The more that the two groups can let go of their 'noble self-image" and begin to collaborate the more likely it will be that trust can exist.

## Provider and the Pharmaceutical Industry

Providers have a long standing and multi-faceted relationship with the pharmaceutical industry. The relationship goes back as far as the 1800s. Like today, the pharmaceutical industry worked to educate physicians regarding new medications such as morphine and insulin. Like most other interactions, the relationship and associated trust depends on the context of the association. There is a relatively small group of health care providers that have deep relationships with the industry due either to their partnerships in drug discovery or their involvement in clinical trials of new medications.

These providers have partnered with the pharmaceutical industry in identifying better treatments to care for their patients. The large portion of providers have a more limited relationship through their interactions with pharmaceuticals representatives.

For a period, there was belief that the relationship between the manufacturers and the providers was based on pens, meals, and trips, all forms of potential conflict of interest. Interestingly, for the most part, this was not the case. For many years, the pharma reps were considered educators. Medications have become foundational in the treatment of both acute and chronic medical conditions. Seventy-five percent of provider visits include the prescribing of at least one medication. The widespread use of medicines requires healthcare providers to stay current on medication options and usage. Much of the education that providers receive about medicines has been found to come from three sources: national meetings, journal articles and pharmaceutical representatives. If providers are relying on the drug representatives to educate them about their medications, are they trusting the right person? In 2003, more than half of the $1.4 billion dollars spent on accredited continuing education in the U.S. was funded by commercial sources. (Moynahan, Drug company sponsorship of education could be replaced at a fraction of the cost. BMJ. 2003, 326, pp 1163) This raises concerns about the provider trusting the information that they are receiving as part of the continuing medical education. A study presented in JAMA showed that 11% of the 103 statements made by the manufacturer were inaccurate, with all the inaccuracies being favorable to that drug company. Unfortunately, when the providers in the room were questioned only 26% were able to recall any of the inaccuracies. (Ziegler M. 1995).

> Dr Solo is a cardiologist. He shared with us that as a specialist, all his patients are on at least one medication with many of them on five or more. For many years, he saw drug representatives in his office on Tuesdays. "They would bring lunch and share with us information on heart disease and the medications that their company was distributing. Did I trust what they told me? Did I feel obligated to prescribe their medicines.? First, all the companies came to the office. This evens the field. Secondly, it is my job as a doctor to make sure that

the information that I am getting from them is true. They are only one source of information. My career is worth more than a meal or a sleeve of golf balls. I trust myself. I cannot say that this is true for all doctors."

It was not unusual for a pharmaceutical representative to integrate the education and information that they were sharing with healthcare providers with the giving of objects of some value. A study done in 2012 found that 84% of US providers received some type of payment, gift, meal, travel or free sample from the pharmaceutical industry. The industry has been said to have spent over $27 million dollars on marketing to providers. (Pew Prescription Project 2014) This activity of material giving created concern that providers were being unduly influenced by the manufacturers. In 2002 a voluntary code of conduct between physicians and the pharmaceutical industry was implemented. This codified the exclusion of most gifts, meals and trips offered to providers from the industry. This code of conduct preceded the Sunshine Act of 2010. As part of the Affordable Care Act, CMS put into place the Sunshine Act which requires the pharmaceutical manufacturers to publicly report any gifts, payments and other activities of value over $10 dollars.

Gifting to those with buying power or the "power of the pen" rarely creates a bribery scheme whereas the provider feels an obligation to prescribe in a manner that they would not otherwise do. Most of the providers we spoke to stated that receiving "tchotchkes" or gifts from the manufacturers did not influence their decision- making process. Studies have come down on both sides of the argument. Overall, providers are ethical professionals that want to do what is best for their patients. They look to the scientific evidence and their peers to act in an appropriate manner. The problem is that even if this is not the case, there is a perception that this could be true. Are providers putting their professionalism on the line? Do their actions risk losing the trust of their patients? Interestingly, when asked whether it would matter to their patient as to whether they received gifts from the manufacturers, 51% of patients say they are not sure that it would matter but they would at least want to know about it. Over 50% of individuals went on to say that they would trust both the pharma industry and their doctors less if their doctor accepted gifts. (Green et al, 2012)

For the most part, gifts to providers are a thing of the past. Some of the education and support that providers received from the pharmaceutical manufacturers were outside of the traditional medication detailing model. Many manufacturers were offering more general education on topics such as the "The Business of Medicine", "Value Based Contracting" or "Engaging your Patient's in their own Healthcare." Lack of trust and concern over the manufacturer's potential undue influence has created a void in some of these topics, especially for young physicians.

> Dr Patel is a 45-year-old pediatrician who shared his story. "I was a chief resident in pediatrics and was given the opportunity to attend a three- day educational event by a pharma company. The entire focus was a primer on the business of medicine. I had spent three years on learning the science and practice of pediatrics but had never been given any information on what I needed to know about basic business principals. The team that taught us were three pediatricians that had gone into three different types of medicine. It was great. Drugs were never discussed. Did I feel obligated to use that manufacturers products? Not for a moment. That was not the point of the seminar. In fact, I don't even remember who the company was. It is a shame that these types of programs are no longer offered."

The last 30 years has brought significant changes to healthcare. Many of these changes have had both direct and indirect implications for healthcare providers. The degree of which providers trust others and how providers are trusted has been affected. For healthcare to achieve its desired goal, healthcare providers need to remain diligent around issues of trust.

## Health Plan and Trust

"We aren't perfect. When we screw up, we have to own it and not make excuses. We work every day to maintain and regain trust"
Mark Ganz, CEO Regence Health Solutions

Aligned goals are an important factor associated with trust. It is rare that the financial gain of one entity on the back of another entity is a shared goal. How often do we hear that Health Plans only care about money? Interestingly, economics were the impetus for forming most health insurance companies. With few exceptions, the United States healthcare system and associated insurance model is based more on a financial opportunity for employers and hospitals. Access of care for consumers became an outcrop of this opportunity. That is not to say that clinical care played no role. In a few cases, the formation of the health insurance company allowed for individuals to receive care for illness and injury that they otherwise would not be possible. One such example is the Pierce County Medical Bureau. The Pierce County Medical Bureau was founded in 1917 by timber workers in the pacific northwest. The group pooled their wages in order to create a fund that would pay for the care of participating loggers that were hurt or injured. This, the first pre-paid model, paved the way for health insurance in the U.S. Eventually, this organization became Regence Blue Cross of Washington. This began a slow but steady pattern of workers organizations and unions coming together in order to fund pre-paid health insurance for their workers. Like the timber workers in Washington state, teachers in Dallas, Texas formed such a group in 1929. The insurance was created in partnership with Baylor Hospital with all the care being received at Baylor. Once again, the insurance was focused predominantly on illness and accident- based care.

Additional employer- based health insurance organizations began to arise utilizing the pre-paid model similar to Pierce County Medical Bureau and the Baylor Pre-Paid Teachers Insurance Plan. (Interestingly, both these early pioneers became Blue Cross Blue Shield Plans) or an indemnity type plan which paid for the services past service delivery. The next expansion of health insurance occurred during World War 2. Labor constraints due to the war created significant competition for manpower and because of this the National War Labor board created the Stabilization Act of 1942. This law allowed for the government to freeze salaries in order to address the increasing need of labor and reduce the risk of inflation. To attract workers, companies began offering health insurance instead of increasing wages. In addition to this employer inducement program, employers were also given tax breaks associated with these health insurance plans. By 1960, a growing number of individuals had some form of health insurance through their employers. There remained a number of poor or elderly individuals who were not covered by the employer- based health insurance system. In 1965 President Johnson signed the Medicare and Medicaid programs into law in order to address this gap in availability of health insurance. The Medicare and Medicaid Act was the first real expansion of health insurance outside of the private sector. For the most part, most health insurance plans were a financial instrument that was limited to a focused portion of healthcare. During this time, consumers had a congenial and trusting relationship with health care insurance companies. These organizations help to fund care that had previously been paid for by the consumer.

Prior to the 1950's health insurance covered care for the ill or injured. There was little attention focused on preventative healthcare. One exception to this model was Kaiser Permanente. Like the Pierce County Medical Bureau, The Permanente Health Plan was based on a pre-paid model. A number of unions in the California area found this type of plan to be both affordable and aligned with the union's goals. In 1951, The Permanente Group began offering preventative screening.

The Permanente group was one of only a few organizations that included these services until the HMO Act of 1973 (The Act). The Act was created through the advice of Dr Paul Ellwood in order to address the rising costs of healthcare. The Act is impactful for five reasons; first is that it provided money to create a new form of health insurance, the Health Maintenance Organization (HMO). Secondly, the HMO act was the first time that a health insurance model was being created with the primary purpose of cost savings. Third, the newly formed HMO model encouraged the promotion and coverage of preventative health care services in addition to the services that had previously been covered by health insurance. Ellwood and his proteges believed that keeping people healthy through prevention would lower health care costs. The fourth factor tied to the Act was that this was the first time that health insurance interacted beyond the simple focus of paying a bill for covered services. This model created an interaction that utilized tools that reviewed and interacted with the provider and the consumer in order to impact both healthcare costs and quality. Thus, began the transition of the industry from "Health Insurance Plan" to "Managed Care." The fifth significant factor created by the Act was the move of health care from a not-for-profit model to a for profit model.

---

Impact of HMO Act of 1973

1. Funding for new insurance Model (The HMO)
2. Created to cost contain
3. Coverage of preventative care
4. Oversite of care
5. Move from not-for-profit insurance

---

The HMO model of care focused on three areas: prevention services, utilization oversight by the organization with an emphasis on the traditional acute and chronic services and a new focus on quality of care.

Although many of the techniques that were created as part of the HMO model, especially those concentrating on the utilization management, were adopted by some of the more traditional health insurance plans, it was the HMO that received the greatest attention and pushback. This was the first time that the consumer experienced a third party interjecting themselves into the physician/patient relationship. No one likes to be told that they cannot have what they want or need. These actions by the health insurance companies, especially the HMOs lead to a significant increase in anger and distrust of the healthcare system. The backlash by consumers and providers was regularly shared on the nightly news and became the fodder for many movies and television shows including John Q and "As Good as It Gets." Many of the stories focused on the withholding of services in order to both save money as well as generating significant profits for the shareholders of the for-profit health plans. The destruction of trust during this time for healthcare in general and the HMO industry in specific created lasting scars for the industry.

What is rarely discussed is the improvement of access and quality of care that the consumer enjoyed during this time. The use of evidence-based guidelines for conditions such as asthma, diabetes and heart disease, preventative care services such as developmental visits and immunizations for children and chronic illness and cancer prevention services for adults all were tracked and paid for by the HMO. It was the first time with the exception healthcare insurance through Kaiser Permanente that these activities were paid for. This insurance model should have created a positive relationship between the insurance industry and the consumer and in under other circumstances probably this good will would have increased trust. Unfortunately, educating, supporting and paying for these positive activities were not the things getting the attention. During the few instances in which this information was shared by the HMO organizations or The National Committee for Quality Assurance (NCQA) which oversaw these activities beginning in 1991, many people were hesitant to believe the information due to their lack of trust in the HMO system.

Johanna is a mother of four. She lived in a three- generation home with her children, her husband and her husband's parents. While her children were growing up. Johanna worked for the local school district and received her family's healthcare through her job. Johanna shared that she was initially very concerned that her family would not receive the care that she needed due to the fact that her health insurance was through an HMO. Johanna went on to say that all my children's visits and shots were covered through this insurance. Initially, my mother-in- law would get angry stating that she never took her children to the doctor when they were healthy. She felt I was wasting money. I explained to her that this was all paid for by insurance. She did not believe me. It was funny, when she finally understood how this insurance worked, she was amazed."

How much of an HMO or even health insurance company lack of trust is due to real circumstances is unclear? Starting with the advent of HMOs and other forms of managed care insurance we witnessed stakeholders, especially providers and consumers, focus on negative issues such as the withholding of services instead of the positive impact such as increasing preventative care and immunizations. This negative viewpoint created significant level of mistrust. David Shore's book explained that HMO enrollees are less trusting than other insurance plans. A study that he quotes from the Center for Studying Health System Change in 2002 found that only 13% of those surveyed had a "great deal" of confidence in the HMO. There were a number of reasons for these emotions to exist; it was a new model of insurance that many people did not have past experience with, it was during a period of rapid scientific discovery in conjunction with the first time that a third- party had input into a consumer's care and the HMO model was receiving a great deal of negative media coverage. One example that stands out focuses on high dose chemotherapy and autologous bone marrow transplant for women with breast cancer.

During the 1990s more than 41,000 women underwent this difficult procedure with the hope of surviving an otherwise fatal diagnosis of stage 4 breast cancer. During a ten -year period, health insurance companies, patients and physicians participated in a very public battle of the efficacy and coverage for this treatment protocol. The health insurance plans pointed to the scientific evidence that showed little efficacy in this very costly treatment while the providers and patients articulated that the patient had little to lose. This argument was played out almost daily both in the courts and in the press. These led to a public uprising that has had implications lasting 30 years. Even as on-going science has proven the health insurance plans to be correct in their view that there was no scientific evidence supporting the treatment, health insurance plans continue to struggle to achieve trust by the public. A question was asked a group of individuals: How often do your feel that the health insurance company would hold back cancer care for a child.

1.  26% stated that this occurs often
2.  40% states that this occurs sometimes

Overall, 2/3 patients felt that a health insurance company would withhold needed care. When the individuals were given actual statistics of non-coverage, individuals (both patients and providers) stated that they did not trust the statistics.

The negative reputation and lack of trust of health plans is not unfounded. There are some decisions that a number of health plans, especially the HMOs of the 1990s, made that gave both consumers and providers reasons to be distrustful. One of these actions was the "gag rule clauses" that were included in many providers contracts. Gag clauses restricted providers from discussing certain diagnostic and treatment options with their patients. These clauses were created to limit treatments in order to control costs. In the mid 1990s, the AMA called for the dissolution of these contractual clauses. Although these clauses disappeared in 1996, gag clauses still remained for a period of time in other types of contractual agreements. One example of gag clauses includes the inability of pharmacists to provide drug price information to their customers .This form of gag clause was made illegal in October of 2018. In both the case of physicians being unable to share all treatment options with their patients and pharmacists unable to share pricing information to help to reduce a consumer's out of pocket costs created a situation where trust was reduced between all stakeholders; the individual, physicians, pharmacists, pharmacies, Health plans and PBMS. No one was left untouched.

A consumer's lack of trust in health insurance plans is not universal. In other industries one's own experience can often impact trust.

> Saline is a mother of 6. She shared with me her transition to trust in regard to health insurance. In the 1980's she received her health insurance through her work as a schoolteacher. She had four children and was concerned initially that her children would not receive the care that they needed due to the reputation of the HMO industry as well as not knowing the pediatrician that would be taking care of her children. Having 6 children under the age of 15, all in school, the children were often in the pediatrician's office receiving care for viruses that they contracted as well as injuries common to children, including a broken arm from a jungle gym. Jennifer very quickly learned that the care that she received from both the physician and the health plan were excellent and that her original concerns were unnecessary. In fact, the next year when additional insurance offers were available, she did not go to a more open PPO option. When asked, she shared that she trusted both the insurance company and her children's pediatrician, as "they had done right by her."

The lesson is that experience and a strong interpersonal relationship overcame the bad press and pre-conceived notions.

## Who consumers trust to administer health insurance

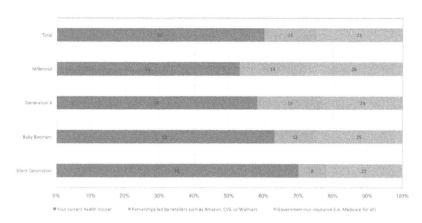

Source: Adapted from Revive Trust Survey, 2017

The HMO Act of 1973 created the move from a not-for-profit model of health insurance to one that is for- profit based. We asked a number of those that we surveyed whether they trusted the not-for- profit more than the for- profit model. The answer to this question varied from those that stated that the profit status of insurance does impact their level of trust to those in which it made very little difference in how they feel or trust the organization. Interestingly, most of those that we spoke to could not identify the profit status of the organization of their health plan. 32% of those that were asked thought that all health plans were for-profit. One individual that we spoke with shared this" No one trusts Amazon, Apple and Volvo less because these companies are publicly traded for - profit companies. Why should the financial model matter? To me, I trust organizations that do what they say they are going to do." Not only does profit status not impact trust, both our study and the Revive 2017 trust survey found that neither providers or consumers see significant difference in the health plans regarding how they are treated and how much they trust the organization. When we shared this information with the health plan executives, they were quite surprised.

It is time to take a moment and turn the table around and ask the question as to whether Health Plan executives trust the consumers that they are responsible for? This question is not easily answered. In most cases, the relationship between a consumer and the health plan is not direct. Over 50% of the time, the health plan's fiduciary responsibility is through the employer or the government. The consumer is limited or has little choice in which health insurance company they utilize. In addition, coverage decisions that appear to be made by the health plan are made by the payer (employer or government). This creates a situation where the health plan has "dual responsibility," the client (payer) and the consumer. This often creates a challenging situation for the health plan.

> Simil, a senior health care executive talked about the impact of this "dual responsibility." I have mixed feelings about the member (consumer). First, I don't think that the member understands the whole health insurance thing. They know that their employer pays for a portion of the premium. They do not know how much the employer is covering in costs. This lack of transparency creates a "story in the members' eyes. All they see is that their costs are going up. Some members feel like they are owed any care that they want. It's similar to someone paying a monthly fee to go grocery shopping. You can go as often as you want and buy whatever you want. They want to go daily and buy filet mignon. Don't get me wrong, I believe most members are good people but just do not understand insurance. At the end of the day, we need to work to cover those things that are appropriate and that members need. We do want to keep them happy"

There is a subset of individuals that have a direct contractual relationship with the member. Those that are buying individual policies for themselves and those that are covered by Medicare or Medicaid are directly choosing their health plan coverage. Health plan executives understand that a lack of trust by these consumers may cost them both in membership as well as in reputation. Although there is very little formal research in how health plan executives feel about their members, a large majority of the executives that we spoke to stated that they trust their members.

> Rica is a retired Healthcare executive. The health plan that she led included a PACE (Program for the Care of the Elderly) program. The individuals that are enrolled in these programs are those that are most frail, community dwelling elderly individuals. Most of these members are dually eligible for both Medicare and Medicaid. During our conversation he shared his experiences with the members and their families. "I often heard our members say that the program was too good to be true. They wanted to know what the catch was. It was not unusual for these people to have organizations make lots of promises and then not fulfill them. Once they experienced the program, they began to trust us. I made it my goal, to change each of the members and their family's minds about who and what we are. I understand that we can only be successful in helping them if they trust us"

Like the quote from Mark Ganz, " We work every day to maintain and regain trust". Overall, what we heard from the health plan executives was that regardless of the type of insurance, they work to support their members to the best of their ability.

The health plans relationship with providers is another area of great importance. We spoke earlier about the lack of trust of providers to the health plans. What do health plans executives feel about the providers within their network? Do they trust them? The 2017 Revive Health Trust Index showed that health plans have more trust in providers at

67% than doctors or hospitals have in health plans 54%. We found in our survey that the answer is, it depends. Going back to Dr Quints, Mary Filipe and Dr Sally all had areas where they felt that they were "part of the team." Trust begets trust. It has been said that "The only way to make a man trustworthy is by trusting him. And the easiest way to make him untrustworthy is to mistrust him and show your mistrust." This statement is true for the health plan executives that we spoke to. Those executives that felt that the providers goals were aligned to theirs were more likely to trust the provider.

> Rica, the CEO that we heard from earlier shared" providers are always telling us that the health plans create lots of hassle factors for us, the fact is that this is sometimes true. We don't do this on purpose. We are looking to achieve the same goals most of the time. Unfortunately, we have our systems and they have theirs. We need to find a way to sit together and do our best to create a system that achieves those administrative goals along with the ultimate goal, the patient."

The role of the health plan executive also impacted the level of trust that they had. Actions and interactions are the bricks that build a trusting relationship.

> Darma leads the Quality and Utilization Management team at a national health plan. Darma shared her frustration and lack of trust for many of the providers that she interacts with. Some of the providers are reasonable and honest people that really want to help their patients. They are willing to interact with us in a thoughtful and educated manner. Unfortunately, not all of the providers are like this. We do not like to post the guidelines that we utilize for our coverage decisions because it is amazing how many providers will lie in order to achieve their goal. I had one doctor that wrote a letter that the patient absolutely had to have a specific medication because they were allergic

to the medicine that was covered. That is fair and we approved the coverage. The next year, the doctor wrote us a letter for the same patient stating that they needed the first drug because they were allergic to the drug that they were on. This was the same drug that they requested by appeal the previous year. It is possible but unlikely that this was really the situation. This is a provider that I will have trouble trusting in the future."

Lou is the Director of Provider Networks for the same health plan. Lou shared his feelings and level of trust for providers. "I have to negotiate with these individuals every day. You would think that I would not like or trust these people. Sure, they are looking to get the best contract possible. The truth is that most of them are reasonable. I actually respect that they are good negotiators. Sure, there are a few that are jerks but for the most part, these are professional individuals and therefore I trust them."

As these examples clearly show, trust of the health plan executive for the providers that they deal with depends on their interactions and experiences. Many of those within the Health Plan that focus on quality or utilization management feel that it is their role to protect the member by addressing quality deficits in care through potential lack of a physician following scientific evidence, or even fraudulent practices that maximize the providers revenues. A common perception is that health insurance companies have control over doctors and that their "imposing their will" has decreased the quality of care. The reality is that managed care in conjunction with the employers that contract with them, had been early adopters of quality programs such as NCQA. Through these focused initiatives the health plans have improved the quality in a number of areas including childhood immunizations, use of correct medicines for heart failure after hospitalizations, and care for people with diabetes.

The relationship between a health insurance plan and a provider has been primarily focused on a payment arrangement; what will the doctor be paid for giving care to the patient that has the health plan insurance? In addition to payment, the contractual relationship allows the provider access to patients that are covered by the health insurance plan through the provider network. This is a model that has been in place for more than 35 years. The relationship between the health plan and the provider is going through a number of changes. The payment arrangements are changing, and this is creating the opportunity to change the trust equation between the two stakeholders. Over the last few years an increasing number of providers have become employees of a health plan. One example of this is United Healthcare, which is presently the largest employer of physician practices in the United States. Many other providers remain independent from the health plans. Their relationship continues to be based on contractual arrangements. Even with these providers, the contractual arrangements are evolving into one that tries to align the goals of the two stakeholders.

Contractual relationships are changing as well. The contract between a health plan and the provider has historically been based on a payment for services model. A provider was paid on a fee schedule model. In addition to the fee that the provider would receive, there would often be an incentive bonus attached to either quality and/ or utilization metrics. These type of payment models often created dis-aligned incentives. If you are paid to do more, it is human nature to do more. We as humans do what we are rewarded for. This is not to say that all providers engage in services for the sake of payment only. In fact, this is not the norm of most providers. Unfortunately, the bad actions of a few create distrust in the many. The Medicare Provider Utilization and Payment Database was created in 2012 and began public disclosure in 2013.This database created transparency in payments that individual doctors were receiving from Medicare. What became clear quickly after being published was that there were a number of providers that were making outsized income associated with Medicare in ways that were difficult to explain. This shed a light on a number of those that were dishonest in both action and billing. Unfortunately, it created a level of distrust broadly across the industry including in the health plans.

> Debbie is a 45-year-old healthcare executive. In discussing the issue of trust within her industry shared her thoughts with me. She shared that there is all this talk about "value- based care and value -based contracts between payers and providers. My question is value to whom? This is the payers passing on risk to providers and providers seeing this as a way to gain back control and receive more money. No one is talking about the impact on value to the patient. This is why I do not trust the industry as a whole.

Many of the volume -based payment model contracts also included incentives associated with quality. This created interactions that bred distrust such as arguments over the metrics associated with quality. During my time as a consultant, I often found myself sitting with a provider group discussing quality contracts and payments. My advice to the providers was consistently that "you need to know your metrics better than the health plan does". Follow them, early and often. If you see that your quality metrics are low, address them. Put a quality plan together." It is not unusual for a provider group to not collect their own quality metrics and then find themselves at the negotiating table with the health plan that tells them that their quality is not high enough to attain the incentive bonus. Health care providers are similar to the inhabitants of Lake Wobegon. They believe that they are all above average. When they hear that they are not, they get angry and feel that the health plan is looking to cheat them. This creates a level of mistrust. On the other hand, the health plan loses trust in the provider for trying to "game" the system. The good news is that this situation is occurring less often as the health plans are providing quality metrics to the providers on a regular basis so that it is less often the case that the providers are surprised by their metrics. That being said, there was one Health Plan executive that said, "if I had a dollar for every doctor that told me that the data was wrong and that they did not make their quality incentives because their patients are sicker than other doctors, I would own my own Island."

Some interesting factors from the qualitative portion of the survey include the concerns over heath plan consolidation and the power that the consolidation gives the plan over others including providers, hospitals and health systems. This has created an increased lack of trust and difficulties in negotiating contracts. The contractual arrangements between health plans and providers are changing. Over the last several years, health plans recognized the importance of finding mutual ground with physicians. One way this is being achieved is through the change in focus of the contractual arrangement between the two stakeholders. Volume -based contracts have begun to be replaced by those that focus on patient goals and outcomes. A Sullivan Cotter report found that value-based contracts increased by 5-7% from 2018-2019, with 62% of organizations incorporating some type of value-based contracting for providers.

The more traditional payment for volume or fee for service model, created a system that is not only unsustainable but also does not align the goals of the stakeholders. Tying payment for patient outcomes allows providers to utilize their knowledge and skill in order to achieve what health plans and consumers hope is the ultimate goal. For providers that contract with health plans in this manner, the utilization-based oversight and scrutiny that has occurred since the late 1980s will be replaced. Physicians have seen this type of oversite as one of the major drivers in creating distrust between the two stakeholder groups.

Utilization activities will not disappear overnight but will decrease over time in conjunction with greater use of value -based contracting.

The alignment of the two groups on high level quality care focused on goals and outcomes has the opportunity to create a partnership and a win-win situation.

The world in which health plans have existed has changed over the last forty years. The contractual relationships that they have had with providers is one of those changes. Up until the last few years, health plans contracted with physicians that were either in solo practice or in groups. Today about 90% of positions offered to newly graduated physicians are through employment to a larger organization including health plans. In all, almost 70% of family physicians are employed and have no ownership stake in the practice. Many of the employment positions are in conjunction with Health Plans. United Health Care alone, employs more than 50,000 physicians. Andrew Witty, the CEO of United Healthcare stated in a Beckers' Interview on September 17, 2019 that by employing physicians, his organization can offer the highest quality of care for it's members. "We have a platform from which we can envision a different type of environment and care. What we are aiming to do here is look at every step of the journey for patients from diagnosis to a cure…We want to straighten out the incentive system and make sure patients and physicians have the right information." Although United Healthcare employs more health care providers than any other health plan, others have a similar vision, better care for the consumer in a more integrated fashion. It is not unusual to hear some people say that Health Plans can have more control over these providers through an employment model. We found that a large number of providers that are employed by health plans are satisfied with the relationship. It may be that there is selection bias, providers that have remained employed are those that are most satisfied. Those that are unhappy leave to seek employment in other venues. How do health plan executives perceive their provider peers?

Jim is a health plan executive that is responsible for the Provider division of the health plan. "The reality is that providers are employees like the rest of us. We expect them to do their job caring for our members. Yes, we trust them. It is our job to give them the tools to be productive and meet the company goals, it is their job to practice good evidence- based medicine. "

To date, there have been no studies that compare trust between health plans and providers that are employed by the health plans and those that are not. If a common purpose and aligned incentives are an important factor in trust, this type of relationship may help to build new trust bridges.

How do Health Plan executives feel about hospitals and hospital systems? Like physicians, hospitals interact with Health Plans through contractual arrangements. Historically, the relationship has tended towards being antagonistic as the hospitals want to be paid as much as possible, while the health plans want to pay them as little as possible.

> Emilio is the Chief Operating Officer of a regional health plan. "The hospitals are always looking for us to bail them out financially. Four dollars for a Band-Aid, really? Costs and billing would be their problem except for the fact that our members come to us complaining about how much they have to pay. The recent argument seems to be cost inequality and facility fees. It should not cost three times more for a member to get an x-ray at the hospital than at a free-standing radiology center or a member seeing a doctor at a primary care clinic owned by the hospital."

Virginia Hite in a May 22, 2020 article wrote about some unique ways previous competitors and adversaries are beginning to form unique relationships due to their experiences during the Covid 19 pandemic

1.  Alignment on standards of care
2.  Sharing of pertinent data

3. Cross stakeholder committees
4. Aligned goals with financial commitments

In addition to these types of initiatives, some health plans are partnering with hospitals to form new health insurance companies. Health Plans will have to begin to heal wounds and build bridges. Past distrusts have to be overcome in order for these types of activities to be successful.

Up until now, we have focused on relationships and trust issues between the health plans and fellow stakeholders. These relationships don't tell the whole story. Healthcare executives often forget the importance of trust within their organizations. This is true whether these executives lead hospitals, health systems or health insurance organizations. Employees of each of these organizations need to act as ambassadors for their organizations. In order for this to occur they must trust in both the organization as a whole as well as trusting the leadership of the organization acting in a manner that supports the goals and responsibilities of the organization as well as supporting each of the employees of the organization. This is especially true of younger employees that are often driven by mission.

As we discussed in the patient and provider sections, discordance between race, gender, cultural and religion of individuals has the potential to create trust issues. These underlying demographic discordances of traits manifests to impact trust in the workplace.

# Levels of trust between stakeholders

| | Average(Range) |
|---|---|
| Health systems' level of trust in Health Plan | 52.0 (36.3-68.0) |
| Physicians' level of trust in Health Plan | 55.8 (52.8-58.4) |
| Health Plans' level of trust in Health Systems | 59.4 (68.4-75.0) |

**Source: Adapted from Revive Trust Survey, 2017**

August is the CEO of a healthcare services organization. August talks about the fact that he is often one of the very few "Black or Brown individuals" at a meeting or a conference. He believes that others do not consider him a "member of the club" and therefore an outsider. "This distrust has often manifested itself in negotiations that he has had with the Health Plans that he contracts with. The power hierarchy often is skewed away from me. Over time we get to know each other, and this trust diminishes, it never goes away completely."

Taisha, a senior executive for a Health Plan stated that as the only female, the lack of gender diversity in her fellow executives creates a trust challenge for her. This lack of trust is exemplified in two ways. She shared that she is often treated as a diversity hire and her contributions are often disregarded. She also explained that lack of diversity impacts how the other executives perceive the individuals that they serve. "The lack of knowledge that diverse groups bring to the table creates a sort of "diversity competence" to those they serve. How do we know what our members may need if we don't have the openness of a diverse team?"

Beyond demographics, actions between individuals within an organization can create or destroy trust.

> Alberta is a senior executive at a large health plan.
> "I attended a meeting of the senior team. This consisted of about 70 people from around the company. We were gathered to review the results of the employee engagement survey. The CEO began the conversation by yelling at the entire team regarding the results. The feedback from the employees focused on how the CEO and the senior leadership was not supporting the employee base. He took no joint responsibility and then went on to say that we were making him look bad. A group of executives got together after the meeting and shared their frustration and distrust of the CEO due to his reaction. "

Alberta's story is a good example of what Don Berwick calls "vertical trust." Vertical trust is the thread of trust that runs from the very senior executives in the healthcare system down to the clinicians and on to the consumer. Only through vertical trust can all stakeholders have aligned goals and positive intention. If there is lack of trust within an organization, this bleeds to external trust of the organization.

Traditional health plans interact with a number of stakeholders. Two influencers of trust that are often overlooked are the government and the media. Both of these stakeholders have a notable history in regard to health insurance companies. We will go into greater depth on these two stakeholders later in the book. The key takeaway is that both government, both state and national, and media, whether more traditional mass media such as newspapers or television, or newer forms of social media have been shown to have a large impact on trust within the healthcare environment. It will be important if we are to change the trust dynamic that these two stakeholders be actively engaged.

Health plans need to be brutally honest with themselves. For over 30 years, the health plans were considered the bully in the school yard. The good news is that more recently, they have realized that it is important to find mutual ground with other stakeholders within the healthcare environment. Reducing activities that create barriers to trust and working towards collaborative interactions will increase the opportunity for healthcare to evolve. Changing the relationship takes time. Trust will have to be regained. The road to trust will require all sides to put aside past experiences and come to the table to communicate. Finding ways to collaborate and respect each other's roles and expertise is a good starting place.

We talked about some of the challenges in the relationship between health plans and hospitals. What happens when a hospital becomes a health plan? This model is not new. Kaiser Permanente is an example, and they are not alone. Geisinger Health Plans Chief Financial Officer, Kurt Wrobel feels that a provider sponsored health plan is the next natural step. Will this transition change the trust dynamic between hospital, the consumers and provider?

## Hospitals/ Hospital Systems and Trust

Before the birth of modern medicine, hospitals were buildings where people went to die. This idea changed in the early 1900s. Because death was the most common outcome, and was expected, trust was not much of a factor. Due to advances in medicine and the advent of antibiotics, hospitals began marketing themselves as places where the ill could get care and heal, a place of safety and comfort. As the century advanced, hospitals realized that they needed to fill their beds. Activities such as childbirth and other life-giving interventions began to occur more often. In 1923, Baylor Hospital found that it needed to identify additional ways in which to keep the hospital financially viable. Baylor identified an opportunity to partner with the teacher's union and offer the hospital's services on a pre-paid basis. Although, like the direct physician contracting model created by

Pierce County Medical Bureau, the Baylor model has been identified as the first hospital to directly contract with an employer to create a health plan aligned with care for the employees of a specific company. In 1957, Kaiser Foundation Harbor Hospital was specifically built for the members of the Longshore and Warehouse Union employees and their families. Once again, a hospital created a model of partnering with the health plan directly associated with an employer. Hospitals were taking an active role in creating and delivering care to consumers. These activities created a positive image "halo" for the hospitals and allowed them to develop trusted relationships with all those that interacted with them.

The last 40 years has brought significant changes to hospitals. Technology has improved and unlike the early years of hospital care, more people are saved by the new capabilities that hospitals offer. Unfortunately, other changes have also occurred. During this time, we have seen an increase in hospital consolidation. These larger more complex organizations addressed many challenges for the hospitals but also created a new challenge, the degradation of trust by other stakeholders. Many perceive these larger hospital system entities as focused largely on their own financial health and less on the health of the consumer. These changes have created rifts in the relationships between hospitals and the stakeholders that they interact with. This previous halo of trust has paled. Sachian Jain MD MBA, CEO and President of Scan Health Plan, stated in a 2021 article in Healthcare Innovation that "many C-suites of hospitals and hospital systems are talking out of both sides of their mouths. They say one thing, but most organizations operate like they're about something else". He goes on to say that although they talk about value based care, they still are relying on the old model of filling up hospital beds.

Trust of hospitals and hospital systems has been challenged by a variety of issues. Many have made headline news across media. Public exposure to the healthcare experience within the hospital system setting, medical errors or financial issues are all being uncovered and discussed daily.

1. Lack in transparency of cost
2. Higher costs compared to similar services at other healthcare facilities
3. Surprise billing
4. Aggressive collections policies
5. Long wait in emergency departments
6. Media coverage of medical mistakes
7. Television and movies where profits are placed over people
8. Public arguments with other healthcare stakeholders
9. Consolidation creating poor consumer experience

As healthcare costs continue to rise at an unsustainable level, fingers are being pointed across the industry. Hospitals have not been immune to their role in the cost equation. In 2018, hospital costs were found to be 33% of the total healthcare spend according to the Kaiser Family Foundation National Health Expenditure data. This significant portion of healthcare costs has shown a bright light of finances for hospitals. The cost issue has become even more contentious as care that was previously only available within the hospital is now available in other settings at a lower cost. Hospitals are beginning to be challenged by competition that did not exist in the past. Competition for the services that they traditionally offered is cropping up in a variety formats; free standing urgent and emergency services, specialty outpatient centers and hospitals and "hospital at home."

In addition to issues focused on unit cost, lack of transparency of these costs as well as surprise and aggressive billing and debt collection practices add to anger and broad -based distrust of the hospital system. These issues have not just created an emotional response from consumers and state and federal agencies but also from many of the healthcare providers that work for them. The Kaiser Health News reported in September 2019, that some of the physicians at UVA Health System were "outraged" by the fact that UVA hospitals had sued 36,000 patients over a 6-year period in order to receive the payment they believed was owed them. Not only had the hospital system sued these patients, they also had seized wages and savings which caused many families to declare bankruptcy. UVA is not the only hospital to have taken these types of actions.

> Doris has been seeing her doctor for many years for her inflammatory bowel disease. Doris trusts her doctor competence as he is considered one of the best in the country. She also trusts him as he always responds when she is having a flair up of her disease. Doris shares with us that she received her bill for a recent visit to her doctor. The bill not only included the cost of seeing her doctor but also a "facility charge." When Doris reached out to her doctor's office, they apologized and shared that this is the new policy of the hospital. Doris then reached out to the hospital billing department. Their response was that they had to make money somewhere. Doris decided to seek care somewhere where they were less focused on "making money somewhere."

One question that is commonly asked; are all hospitals alike regarding trust from others across the healthcare spectrum. Clark and his co-authors compared one's trust in essential hospitals versus those hospitals that did not focus their services on the underserved. The authors conducted a survey of 1000 patients and caregivers that received services at essential safety net hospitals. One major difference in outcomes between the two hospital types was the overall trust score that the essential hospitals received. The survey found that 80% of those surveyed trusted the essential hospital cohort. The three traits that were found to align with the high level of trust by these individuals included competence, environmental quality and the commitment of the hospital to the patient population that it serves. (Clark, 2020). Outside of that one composite trust score being higher in essential hospitals, all other trust factors and demographics were similar. Higher levels of trust were reported in the older, more financially stable and white male populations. In addition to this demographic profile, additional high trust scores were found in those individuals that covered by Medicare or commercial insurance and utilized the hospital for a scheduled visit.

Regardless of public scrutiny, hospitals, like other areas within healthcare are having to evolve. New forms of competition for more traditional services have prompted hospitals to broaden their services. This expansion of services will require hospitals to interact in new ways for which they have little experience. If hospitals want to succeed in these new endeavors, they will have to improve their trust quotient. In addition to acquiring provider practices, hospitals have begun to offer greater health and wellness services. As hospitals have expanded their roles in the healthcare environment, the issue of trust with patients, physicians and the community has become even more important.

Historically, hospitals deepest relationships have been with providers, primarily physicians. The relationship between hospital and providers has been one of mutual needs; hospitals needed providers to perform services within their walls while providers need the hospital as a site of care. It was a mutual need relationship although they did not really have a common goal. This created affiliation and little else. In addition to a relationship based on mutual need, hospitals utilized physicians as a form of free labor. As part of their staff requirements, physicians were required to take call in the hospital emergency department, intensive care units and delivery room when necessary. They were also asked to participate in hospital committees such as the quality and utilization committees. Much of this work was done with limited renumeration. Over time, providers were increasingly unwilling to participate in these activities. This pushback by medical staffs created a fracture in the previously benign working relationship that the two groups had enjoyed. This created strain for the hospitals. A study published in Health Affairs found that in 2005 46% of CEO of hospital and hospital systems found that the difficult relationship with providers was one of the three most important issues.

During this same period, hospitals costs were rising at alarming rates. One of the variables that influenced costs were medical devices. It is not unusual for a hospital to have to stock multiple similar items in order to please the physicians as each desired a different device. This was especially true for surgeons. These devices, often called physician preference items, were often based on relationships on financial, tenure, technology and support that the physicians had with the device vendors. In response to the significant cost pressure that hospitals found themselves to be under, they began taking control of device inventory. What was a physician decision in the past, now became a hospital decision. Hospitals began limiting the choice of the medical devices that physicians utilized. As physicians lost much of their previous autonomy and power, the relationship deteriorated even further. Animosity ensued and trust was lost. Trust that the hospital will do "right by the physician no longer existed

Over the last few years, the relationship has once again changed. In 2012, only 35,700 medical practices were considered hospital owned, that number has increased to 80,000 practices by the end of 2017. This new employment arrangement is different from the early 1990s when many hospitals entered into employment agreements. Many of those agreements failed due to several reasons including the previous focus on primary care and not medical and surgical specialists as well as the payment model that had been used. This more recent employment model has required the hospital and the providers to sit at the same side of the table and identify the factors that bring value to both stakeholders. It has required a level of trust that neither group has had for the other for quite a while. The providers must trust that the hospital administrators are willing to support them and value them as professionals while the hospital must include providers in decision making.

While hospitals are creating closer and more trusting relationships with some providers, they are finding themselves in direct competition with others. Specialty hospitals are not new. For a number of years these hospitals improved the quality of care given due to the focus of the care. The Medicare Modernization Act (MMA) of 2003 created a moratorium on these types of physician owned specialty hospitals. That moratorium expired in 2005. In addition to MMA, the Stark Laws prohibits physicians from referring patients to health facilities where they have ownership. None the less, there has been an increase of specialty facilities through several ownership models. These new types of hospitals and health facilities have created greater competition for hospitals to attract providers and has decreased the loyalty of physicians to hospitals. It has become a bidding war of sorts. In many cases, control and financial arrangements have replaced trust and respect.

As we have discussed, the provider/consumer trust model was the pre-eminent model in healthcare. The hospital's role focused on providing an acute safety net for the most serious of conditions. Trust between the hospital, the provider and the patient was based on capabilities, competence and the transfer of trust from the physician to the hospital. As healthcare has advanced, becoming more complex, so has the trust relationships involving hospitals and hospital systems. Healthcare providers have long been the conduit between the hospitals and consumers. Hospitals relied on doctors to refer their patients to hospitals and their affiliated services such as radiology centers. Over time, the consumer and the hospital were "tied together" through trust and loyalty. Nina Flannigan and the National Healthcare Trust Index asked 1200 consumers "what impacts your decision when deciding what hospital, you should use? The response was overwhelming more than 74% stated that trust was the most important factor when selecting a hospital." Consumers were loyal to one hospital. It would not be surprising to hear someone say, "Memorial is my hospital." It was often said with pride in one's voice. These were the people that took care of them when they were most vulnerable. They had knowledge and skills that the consumer did not have.

As the loyalty of providers to the hospital has waned and healthcare has begun to organize itself in new models, hospitals have realized that they must create a direct relationship with the consumer. Unfortunately, over the last number of years the trusting relationship between hospitals and consumers is deteriorating. As hospitals have grown, they have become more impersonal and bureaucratic. These organizations do not have a "face," they are a complicated compendium of bricks and mortar. The Institutionalization and bureaucratic layering have created a significant challenge in the trust relationship. (Jellinek M. Erosion of Patient Trust in Large Medical Centers. Hastings Center Report, June 1976. 16-17)

> Jacques is a 67-year-old male that shared his thoughts on trust and health. Jacques has been hospitalized twice. "Trust is not part of the equation between me and the hospital. Hospitals are a necessity, not a nicety." "I trust my physician to tell me what hospital to go to."

As the relationship between the hospital and the consumer is not personal, it is difficult for one to say whether they trusted the hospital or not. In general, hospitals are trusted but they are in and of themselves inanimate objects. Like other areas in healthcare, hospitals are perceived as making decisions based on money by those in the hospital that have control. The reality is that hospitals look at consumers as a means of revenue generation. Whether it is the consumer occupying a hospital bed or utilizing other services offered by the hospital system, without consumers hospitals will fail. The era of loyalty that hospitals enjoyed no longer exists. The evolution of healthcare is creating challenges for hospitals that places them in direct conflict with the experiential expectations enjoy in other areas of their lives.

> Ronald is the CEO of a 12- hospital system. "We understand the importance of the patient. The problem is that they have unrealistic expectations. We are here to take care of them when they are seriously ill. This is not Disney World." When asked about the concerns over cost transparency he shared the following: "Taking care of patients costs a great deal of money. Hospitals must be paid fairly so that we can make new technologies available."

The problem for Ronald and his peers is that consumers are frustrated and angry. Sitting in waiting rooms of emergency departments for hours only to be told by receptionists that you will be seen when they get to you, feeling like you are going through a maze to get to your testing location and having dirty public washrooms are not ways to build trust and loyalty with consumers. One's experience with a hospital can impact the relationship. Like other areas within healthcare trust is based on both competence and experience. One may not be able to define quality in hospital care, but they do substitute their experience. Something simple that has nothing to do with care such as bringing the wrong food or the food is not hot, can create a feeling of dissatisfaction and reduce trust around the entire hospital experience. This is like Robert's story earlier in the book. Robert lost trust in his doctor because of a dirty bathroom.

Hospitals are trying to change this perception. They are organizing themselves in ways that are similar to upscale hotels. Unfortunately, it is not unusual that this is surface cover and many of the other aspects of the hospital have not changed. It is unclear as to whether the redecorating of hospitals has significantly impacted trust in these facilities versus other hospitals. One hospital that worked to make major changes in how they function is Cleveland Clinic. In 2006, the Clinic hired Bridget Duffy MD. as Chief Experience Officer. Her role was to transform the Clinic into a more "patient friendly" environment. Dr Bridget Duffy created an environment where everyone in the organization understood their role in focusing and supporting the patient. This brought a renewed sense of trust from patients and families. It was a lesson to the healthcare industry that in addition to competence, there is an important role of compassion that magnifies that trust that comes with competence. Since that time many hospitals have embraced this belief.

The consumer focus that hospitals have worked to integrate into their business model goes beyond consumer trust and loyalty. It has become a larger financial imperative also due to the Hospital Consumer Assessment of Healthcare Providers and Systems (HCAHPS). This is a CMS mandated patient satisfaction survey for all hospitals focused on adult patients. It is focused on 10 areas of patient experience and is used as part of the payment model for Medicare. Hospitals are incentivized by their HCAHPS score by CMS. In addition to payment incentives, the HCAHPS scores are publicly reported. It is unclear how consumers and providers view the HCAHPS scores. HCAHPS are not the only evaluation system that exists. There are several private and public hospital rating systems. The systems vary in evaluation methodologies and questions asked. Unfortunately, there can be significant variation between each of these scores. The variability creates a great deal of confusion which negatively impacts all the scores. Individuals do not know which to believe and therefore tend to ignore all of them. Conflict and confusion breeds distrust. In addition to the conflicting scores, most of the hospital ratings give the user little deep understanding as to the "why" behind the rating.

Providers and consumers are not the only stakeholders that regularly interact with hospitals and hospital systems. Health insurance plans and the government are important to hospitals as they are the predominant payers for services rendered within the hospital system. Like other provider groups, hospitals and health plans often are found to have a contentious relationship focused predominantly on a monetary interaction. This creates the "across the table" relationship with little in the way of shared mission or vision. Our primary research as well as research done by others has found little trust. As one Health Plan CEO stated "the hospitals want everyone to help them. They feel entitled. I have not given up in hoping to interact with them in good faith. I just go in with my eyes open." My conversation with the hospital CEO was not much different. "They want us to do as much as we can but pay us as little as they can." She went on to say," margins speak for themselves, theirs are in the double digits and ours are in the single digits."

Over the last few years, we have seen some thawing of the icy relationships between the two groups. There are two major reasons for these changes. First is the slow evolution from volume -based payments to value -based payments. This is creating partnerships that did not exist in the past. Executives from the two groups are beginning to sit on the same side of the table and find alignment in value metrics that did not exist in the past. It will take a while to see if these partnerships bring the relationship and in time trust to a more positive level.

> "It's time for the government, the payers and hospitals to
> work together for the future of healthcare…"
> Pam Kehaly, President and CEO of
> Blue Cross Blue Shield of Arizona, 2020

What happens when a hospital becomes a health plan? The second trend that is re-defining the relationship between hospitals and health plans is the move for hospitals to integrate with a health plan. This model is not new. We saw this with Baylor in the 1920s and Kaiser Permanente just a few years later. Since that time a number of organizations such as Geisinger Health System, Intermountain and Advocate Aurora are just a few of the more than 100 such systems across the United States. Geisinger Health Plans Chief Financial Officer, Kurt

Wrobel stated that a provider sponsored health plan is the next natural step. Over the last few years, we have once again seen an increase in either the integration of two existing entities or hospital systems becoming insurers with the hope that this form of health system integration will increase quality while decreasing costs. States such as Wisconsin where the hospital systems, many of which have become integrated over the last few years are now launching their own health plans. Will this transition change the trust dynamic between hospital, the consumers, and providers? This is yet to be seen. The alignment of goals, transparency in cost and everyone feeling that they are being positively impacted will have to occur. Concern has been voiced by consumers, providers, and some governmental agencies that these large integrated systems will just allow for greater power and not impact the system as a whole in a positive manner. The Health Plan CEO that we spoke about earlier shared his feelings about this hospital transition into the health insurance business. "They are just looking to cut us out. They want more control. It allows for steerage into the hospitals." Others have stated that they feel that this new model of integration allows the organizations to have greater bargaining power with other health plans.

Hospitals play a crucial role both in the healthcare system and in our communities. It is not unusual for a hospital to be the largest employer in many cities and towns across the United States. Even in large cities, hospitals can be a supportive and influential partner. University of Chicago partnered with the surrounding community on the south side of Chicago to discuss ways in which they could support community health. By doing so, the University of Chicago Hospitals and the local Chicago community found ways to heal trust issues and create a partnership that shared goals and deepened the relationship. A member of a community organization on the South Side of Chicago said it best. " The hospital is a building; it is real estate. It is the doctors and nurses that care for us. It is up to them to stand with the administration and do what is right. We both need each other."

## Pharmaceutical Services (Pharmaceutical manufacturers, Pharmacists, Pharmacy Benefits Managers, etc.)

> Every drug is a triangle with three faces, representing the healing it can bring, the hazards it can inflict and the economic impact of each. All of us-doctors, patients, regulators, taxpayers, insurers and policy makers-must learn how to balance these three dimensions better if we are to get the maximum benefit from this most common and powerful of all healthcare interventions.

Jerry Avorn MD Emeritus Chair Division of Pharmacoepidemiology and Pharmacoeconomics, Brigham and Women's Hospital

More than $511 billion dollars is spent annually on medications in the United States and the pharmacy benefit is the most utilized healthcare benefit offered to consumers. It is unlikely that there is a family in the United States that is not directly or indirectly impacted by someone in their family taking medicines. Nearly 70% of all consumers have been prescribed at least one medicine annually and almost 74% of all visits to a healthcare provider involves the review or prescribing of medicine. The reality is medicines and pharmacy are major "kitchen table issues", a concern that impacts and challenges the average individual and their family. The impact of medication economics and costs have created an environment of mistrust.

> Serine is a 59-year-old woman. She has had diabetes for 10 years. She lives with her husband who has had high blood pressure for several years, her daughter and 2 grandchildren who both have asthma. In all, Serine and her family fill 11 medicine prescriptions a month. "The medicine thing always confuses me. My doctor writes for a drug. I go to the pharmacy to get it filled. First the pharmacy says that this medicine will make me sick because of another medicine that I am on. Next, they tell me that my benefit says that I cannot have

the medicine that I should get so that I don't get sick. All the sudden I have all these people involved in just getting me the right medicine. I don't know who to trust. The truth is that sometimes I end up not filling my prescriptions because it is just too confusing. We go through this with each of our medicines each month. They should be paying me for all the time and aggravation that it takes. I should not be paying them."

Serine's story is not unusual. We have created a system that is hard to understand and even harder to navigate. Serine's trust in the world of pharmacy services is quite different than Doris. You may remember that we spoke to Doris earlier about her lack of trust in healthcare due to cost challenges. During our conversation with Doris, she did share her trust of medications and those that make them

Doris shared that she was diagnosed with her inflammatory bowel disease as a young adult. "For many years, my inflammatory bowel disease ruled my life. I was always afraid to go out. A few years ago, a new drug came on the market. It changed my life. Now, there is nothing I can't do and nowhere I can't go. The people that invented these medicines are my heroes.

Physicians have been able to better care for their patients through the medicines that the pharma industry has discovered. Theoretically, this interwoven situation between consumers, providers and the pharmaceutical industry, should bring trust between the stakeholders. Unfortunately, this is not always the case.

The interactions associated with medicines are complex. One example of the interdependencies within the pharmacy services world focuses on the opioid epidemic. The opioid epidemic in the US has had a significant impact on trust in healthcare environment in general and the pharmaceutical industry in specific. Although the tip of the spear of the crisis is the pharmaceutical companies, especially

Purdue, many others including physicians, retail pharmacies and patient advocacy groups all had a level of responsibility.

The complexity we see today was not always the case. If you go back to the early twentieth century most medicines were provided by the doctors themselves or local pharmacists. Over the last century the model changed. The services associated with manufacturing, prescribing, and distributing medications have grown more complicated and vary significantly. The consumer feels exploited by all those that are involved in their medications, including those that create them, those that prescribe them, those that dispense them and those that are supposedly helping them to afford them.

> Solomon, a 57-year-old male said it this way, "Everyone has a lobbyist making sure that their best interests are taken care of. The only one that has no one fighting for their best interest is the patient. Everyone is making a dollar off our backs. That is just wrong. "

Each organization and interaction have the potential for creating trust within the pharmacy services environment. It is important to understand the interdisciplinary nature of the medication environment in order to untangle the associated touch points and their impact.

## Pharmaceutical Manufacturers

Medications have impacted both the longevity and the quality of a consumer's life. Who creates and makes medicines? The discovery and manufacturing of medicines is the responsibility of the pharmaceutical manufacturers. It is a source of innovation and the work that they accomplish has saved millions of lives. Their discoveries have allowed many people to lead good and productive lives.

> Albert is a senior executive for a large pharmaceutical company. "I went to medical school with the idea of helping

people. Not long after finishing my residency I was offered a position at a drug manufacturer. At that moment I realized that by choosing this as my life's work, I could impact many more people." "I have worked for three manufacturers during my career. I am inspired by the company that I work for. In the past, I trusted my peers, but I did not always feel that the company was focused on what our impact really could be. With this organization, it is all about the patient." "I trust our organization to do the right thing for the right reasons."

Albert went on to share with me that he is often frustrated by how others perceive the industry. "I realize we are all painted with a single brush. That is unfortunate. Some of this is the industry's fault. We injure ourselves. The problem is that it goes beyond just our own actions. Doctors, patients, and the press do not understand what we do. I don't know how to fix that"

Many manufacturers have been in business for over one hundred years. These organization are known for their expertise in science and ability to discover new drugs. For more than fifty years, the pharmaceutical industry was considered a trusted and important partner in healthcare. We met Dr Solo earlier in the book. He shared with us the importance of pharma representatives as educators and a source of current information on new medications coming to market. While he felt they played an important role in his caring for patients he did not feel that the drug representatives unduly influenced his prescribing habits. Dr. Solo is not alone in this belief. A 2013 Harris poll of physicians found that there was a trusting relationship between providers and the pharma industry. However, it also found that high levels of trust could have the potential to impact provider behavior and an increase in prescribing certain medications.

It was not only the health providers that had a trusted partner relationship with the pharma manufacturers, but this was also found between the manufacturers and health insurance plans as well as employers. Often, many early disease management programs were either developed or funded by pharmaceutical companies and delivered by the health insurance plans. One of the earliest asthma management programs was a partnership between a Schering, Rush Health Plans and First National Bank of Chicago.

The 1980s brought in the era of "blockbuster medications." Drugs such as Lipitor, Prilosec and Prozac created a multi-billion-dollar industry. The race was on. This is not to say that financial success is a bad thing. On the contrary, we all like a success story. Greater innovation leading to improved clinical outcomes should be rewarded. The challenge is that this level of success prompted a greater focus and greater scrutiny on the industry. Unfortunately, the era of blockbuster medications has created behaviors that have not always benefited an industry that once was considered a trusted partner.

## Americans' Views of the Pharmaceutical Industry, 2001-2019

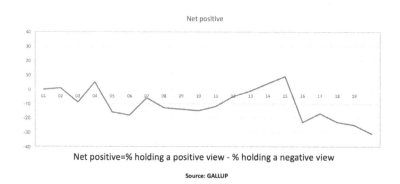

Net positive=% holding a positive view - % holding a negative view

Source: GALLUP

It is unfortunate that an industry that has brought great innovation and changed many American's lives over the last forty years has seen a degradation of trust during the same period. Organizations such as Gallup and Edelman have followed and documented this downward trend. The 2017 Edelman Trust Barometer found that 49% of individuals surveyed were distrustful of the pharma industry. The 2019 Trust Barometer showed a slight increase in trust by 2%. Still not something to be proud of. The September 2019 Gallup poll found that the pharmaceutical companies were last on the trust scale of 25 industries. Even the government was more trusted than the pharma industry. They rated the industry negative 58% of the time and only 27% positively. The other two industries rated at the bottom at 23rd was the healthcare industry and 24th was the federal government. These public opinion polls find pharma was at the bottom of the trust listings for organizations. Manufacturers have been identified as the stakeholder within healthcare that is most responsible for the high cost of care that many are experiencing. Why is this? These are the people that have brought us life altering and lifesaving treatments.

The reasons for the lack of trust in the pharma industry vary but there are five reasons that most commonly cited when discussing the trust challenge that the pharmaceutical industry finds itself in.

---

Reasons for Lack of Trust of the Pharmaceutical Industry

1. Cost of medications
2. Patent litigation
3. Misrepresentation of data and studies
4. Opioid epidemic
5. Misbehavior of leadership

---

## Costs

> "As drug costs began to climb, trust begins to fall.
> They are directly and inversely related."
> Director of Benefits for a Fortune 500 company

Dr C. Everett Koop, the U.S. Surgeon General in 1985 stated that "Drugs don't work in patients who don't take them." His remarks were based on the studies showing the lack of medication adherence in the

United States. "One of the reasons for non-adherence is cost of medications. Do not get me wrong, it is not the only reason. Unfortunately, the high cost of medicines has been in the news since the mid 1980s." During the early time of the HIV era, extremely visual protests occurred both in the United States and abroad against the cost of HIV medicines. People were dying because they could not afford medication. Over time this resolved, and the pharma manufacturers regained levels of trust. Unfortunately, the issue has once again increased and, in some ways, is louder than ever. Drug pricing is considered one of the greatest challenges to trust in the pharma industry today.

The very public conversations regarding increasing costs have decreased the pharmaceutical manufacturers trust level and reputation. During a congressional hearing focused on drug pricing, Mark Alles, the Celgene CEO was asked about the significant rise in cost of Revlimid, a medication used for cancer. Over a 15 year period (2005 to 2019), the drug rose in cost from $215 dollars to $763 dollars. During this time, there was no change in either the formulation or the outcomes associated with the medication. Celgene is not alone in these types of cost increases. A recent survey found 88% of consumers feel that the pharmaceutical company is the major factor for rising health costs. (Physicians Foundation) Chris Lo in his article, The People vs Big Pharma stated, "Drugs should be priced to maximize public health, not to maximize profit." (Lo Chris. The People vs Big Pharma; tackling the industry's trust issues. Pharmaceutical Technology. August 20, 2018.) This is something we heard during many of our interviews. The Pharmaceutical Research and Manufacturers of America (phRMA) states that it costs about $2.6 billion dollars to develop a new medicine. Finding new medicines is not easy. It is time consuming. No one has pushed back on these facts. The question that remains is what is a fair profit for a pharmaceutical company? Many in the U.S. hear that those that live in other countries pay significantly less than those in the U.S. What a consumer knows is that in many cases, they cannot afford their medicines. What good is a medicine that no one can afford to take? This issue has become increasingly heated as new very high-cost medicines come to market, insurance designs such as high deductible health plans have become more prominent, and the negotiating methods between employers, insurance companies, PBMs and manufacturers negatively impact the consumer. Drug costs, like most health care costs, have created a situation where all the organizations blame each other. The pharmaceutical company's counterargument is that without the money that they are charging, innovation for new medications would cease to exist. They also state that the rebate model is not a model that they created. Whether this is true or not, the manufacturers are in a position to take a leadership role in changing the model.

Donald is a CEO of a pharma company. In speaking with Donald, he voiced his frustration about medication costs. He agreed that the industry should be more conscious of price increases but at the same time he shared his beliefs that rebates cloud the issue. He does not understand why rebates remain. He articulated his view that some of the frustration found in patients should be directed to employers and health insurance companies for taking rebates and not passing those on directly to the consumer. He articulated his distrust of "payers" (in this case "employers and health plans") for confusing the issue and placing the blame on the manufacturers. Meanwhile the group with little control over this situation is the consumer. As they stay on the sideline watching this fight, they end up trusting none of the parties involved.

It is not just about the cost of medications; it is also about the lack of transparency associated with drug costs. For pharma companies to have their drug listed on drug benefit formularies, they pay a rebate to the PBM or health plan. That rebate is shared across the PBM and the payers (health plans, employers and governmental entities) that they represent. The amount of the rebate and what is included is often not disclosed. This lack of transparency breeds lack of trust as well. Unless drug payment levels are reformed, there will be increased lack of trust in the pharmaceutical industry.

**Patent litigation-**it has been said that no industry has undergone greater scrutiny for anti- competitive behavior than the pharmaceutical industry. The trust that society and those that are in healthcare give to the pharmaceutical industry for discovering new drugs has been chipped away due to regularly reported anti-competitive behaviors. The drug patent system was created to reward the pharma companies for their great science and hard work in discovering new drugs. Unfortunately, the patent system is also being used to manipulate the very system that it was created to protect. The public has witnessed brand companies trying to retain patent protection or paying generic companies to stay out of the market in order to maximize profits. It is not just the brand companies that have created distrust across the healthcare environment, generic drug companies have also participated in activities that decrease trust. In May 2019, a lawsuit was brought by 40 states attorney generals regarding price fixing activities by generic drug manufacturers. All of these activities are being played out in the courts and in the media creating an aura of distrust of the industry.

**Misrepresentation of data and studies-** Over the last ten years there have been a number of instances where pharmaceutical fraud, or the misrepresentation of data and false statements by the pharma industry has been front page news. Manufacturers must receive FDA approval before a new drug can be released in the market. As part of this approval process, manufacturers are obligated to undergo rigorous testing and analysis. The results of this testing are presented to the FDA so they may assure safety and efficacy of the new drug on behalf of the consumer. In most cases, this process is done appropriately. On rare occasions manufacturers have mis-represented, omitted or falsified the research data. The bad behavior of these few instances has painted a poor picture for the entire industry. Each of these instances create a trust crater that the industry has to climb out of.

**Misbehavior** Harvard Business Review calls it "the scandal effect." Corporate scandal and poor behavior on the part of a senior executive hurt both the company that the individual represents as well as the industry that the company is a member of. 2015 was a bad year for the pharmaceutical industry due to the bad behaviors of two organizations, Valeant and Turing Pharmaceuticals. Valeant was found to have a secret relationship with Philidor, another pharmacy company. Turing Pharmaceuticals CEO Martin Shkreli was arrested for stock fraud after a very public episode of price gouging. Shkreli raised the price of a decade old drug that is used to treat a rare form of muscular dystrophy. To make matters worse, this was not the first time that Shkreli had been in the press This is not the first time he has acted in this manner. Several years earlier, as the founder and CEO of Ovation Pharmaceuticals for increasing the price for a drug that focused on premature infants. He was vilified. Actions like Valeant and Turing create a perception that this type of activity is common across the industry. Whether this is true or not, perception is reality and trust has been scarred.

## Opioid Crisis

One of the most well-known and egregious actions of misbehavior created a crisis that has cost trillions of dollars and many hundred thousand lives across the United States, the opioid crisis. Much of the blame for this public health crisis has been centered on the pharma industry. The opioid crisis has pulled back the covers on how an industry can manipulate the sales and usage of medications. This has created further distrust in the industry. Purdue Pharmaceuticals and other manufacturers created marketing machines that increased the use of pain medications across large groups of individuals, downplayed the risks associated with these medications and created a prescriber pool that was ridiculed as "opiophobias" if those prescribers articulated concerns of addiction and abuse. Oxycontin, a pain medication that was created to treat pain for consumers with cancer, became the poster child for inappropriate corporate influence. Purdue Pharma was not the only manufacturer to participate in aggressive promotional strategies. The courts have found others such as Johnson and Johnson, Insys, and others have also been shown to participate even knowing that the drug was being utilized in dangerous ways. These organizations broke the trust compact that they had with the public through their inappropriate behavior.

Recent opportunities have offered the pharmaceutical industry an opportunity to regain some of the trust that lost over the last few decades. The COVID 19 crisis of 2020 has placed the industry in a position to re-establish themselves as innovators at a time where the country is looking for science to lead us out of a pandemic. The industry's organizations such as PhRMA and individual manufacturers have been front and center in speaking about stepping up front as a leader in fighting the virus through drug discovery and research. Pfizer put forth an ad in April 2020 that stated that they were "taking our science and unleashing it." A Harris Poll in May 2020 about 2 months into the pandemic found that 40% of Americans surveyed stated that pharma had improved its reputation since the beginning of COVID. It is felt by that group that the industry has stepped up and used its resources to help with the response of the outbreak. This includes tests, treatment and most recently vaccines. Edelman released a Trust Barometer spring update. This spring survey found that the virus did have an impact on trust levels within the healthcare environment. The survey found that 73% of those that they spoke with expressed trust in the pharma industry. There are still many who see this activity by pharma as an additional revenue opportunity. It will be up to pharma to be sensitive to the pricing models utilized for these discoveries.

A September 2020 Harris Poll found that 40% of those questioned have an improved level of trust in the pharmaceutical industry. Overall trust in the industry was found to be 71% in general, a same number (71%) trust the manufacturers that are actively working on identifying a vaccine for COVID. The positive viewpoint has been found to be driven by three demographic groups; those that live in urban areas (49%), Gen Z and millennials age groups (44%).

---

**Impact of COVID on Trust for the Pharmaceutical Industry**

58% increase due to efforts to develop a vaccine
56% increase due to efforts to develop or find a treatment
56% increase due to efforts to create diagnostic tests
46% increase due to efforts to create protective gear

Harris Poll September 2020

---

Although COVID 19 has placed the conversation regarding cost of medications on the backburner for now, it still impacted the responses of some of the surveyed population. The majority that stated they had a negative level of trust in the pharmaceutical industry (53%) said that the manufacturers should do more to lower the cost of medications that the U.S. public needs. This group's feelings around trust in the manufacturers was found to be based on either public media or social media. Interestingly, those that stated that they had high levels of trust in the pharmaceutical industry were also based on media. This group stated that pharma advertising impacted their positive trust sentiment.

Going forward the question is whether the pharma industry will maintain the levels of trust that they have gained during the pandemic. Much of this will be up to the industry. Can the industry redress some of the actions that created the low levels of trust? Have they over-promised? Can they help to address the cost and access issues that have weighed heavily on certain communities especially those of lower socio-economic status or those of different cultures or races? Can they provide information that can be trusted and not just information that benefits the industry itself? Raising their trust level may require the pharmaceutical industry to measure themselves in different terms. Today, they are measured by the revenues associated with medication sales. This is at a time when breakthrough drugs are being found to treat and cure conditions that previously had no real treatment options. What if they started to measure themselves against clinical or humanistic outcomes? Organizations speak about being consumer centric, unfortunately they have placed themselves in the center of a payment scheme that lacks patient centricity. Just as other areas of healthcare are moving from volume to value, pharma needs to begin their evolution towards this goal. Pharma and health plans have slowly begun to create relationships based on outcome-based contracting. What if pharma were to partner with providers and patients to identify those specific patients where the medication is most likely to work and least likely to cause side effects or complications from the medication. These would be steps in the right direction. During their quarterly earnings calls they do not start with how many heart attacks were reduced or how many people with Multiple Sclerosis no longer are bedridden or on disability, they still start with their success in selling medications. This emphasis increases a desire to sell medications whether needed or not. It is a set up for distrust. It is time that they revise their value statement to one that all stakeholders can appreciate.

## Pharmacists

We all know a pharmacist. They work at the pharmacy at the corner of our street. If you are old enough, they may have even sold you perfume for Mother's Day, and candy after school. The one thing we all have experienced is that they were someone we went to for health care advice. I had my first job at 14 (yes, I was child labor at the approval of my parents) at a local pharmacy. This was the early 1970s. The Hubbard Woods Pharmacy in suburban Chicago was a center of the neighborhood for friendship and advice. The pharmacist that owned the store was a trusted member of both our community and the healthcare community. The pharmacy profession has gone through many iterations in its history. The Edict of Federich the Second in 1240, separated pharmacy from medicine for the first time and created the pharmacy profession. At that time, the role of prescriber and dispenser were identical. The era created four types of pharmacies, the dispensing physician, the apothecary shop, the general store and the wholesale druggist. Wholesale druggists and apothecaries created the chemicals and was the basis for the pharmaceutical manufacturers of today. The Philadelphia College of Pharmacy was founded in 1821. This is the first known pharmacy organization in the U.S. (Yeung Eugene, Pharmacists Becoming Physicians: For Better or Worse? Pharmacy. September 2018)

By the end of the 19th century prescribing physicians became less likely to dispense medications and the role began to further differentiate. For many years the prescribing of medicines and the dispensing of the prescriptions were done by separate entities, the prescriber and the pharmacy, with only a few exceptions. Over the last few years there has been a small uptick in providers also dispensing medications in order to improve medication adherence.

While the historical trend of a merged prescriber and dispenser has changed so has the model of the separate apothecary and general store. Over the last 60 years, the apothecary shop and the general store merged into a single entity, the retail pharmacy. General stores have transitioned to organizations such as CVS, Walgreens, Bartells and single independent pharmacies such as Hubbard Woods Pharmacy all the way up to national chains that sell everything from tires to prescriptions at stores such as Walmart, Target and Costco. While this is the dominant model of retail dispensing, over the last 20 years, we have seen a resurgence of small compounding and dispensing pharmacies that focus solely on the medications and sell little else.

Both small pharmacies and large national chains have recently partnered with community organizations in order to support local health and healthcare events. This has been especially true in underserved Black, Brown and other underserved communities. Retail pharmacies have worked with trusted community organizations such as houses of worship, the beauty and barber shops and community organizers. The transfer of trust from these long -trusted organizations to partnering retail pharmacies have brought health fairs, health education classes and screenings to communities where these services were often not available. The Smidt Heart Institute at Cedars-Sinai in Los Angeles combined the use of clinical pharmacists and 52 black owned barbershops in the Los Angeles area in order to reduce the risk of heart attack and other heart diseases. When individuals came to the barbershop either for a haircut or comradery, they were offered the opportunity to meet with the pharmacist. This allowed for the trust of the barbershop and a center for the black community to transfer the trust within the community to pharmacists that otherwise may not have been trusted. This is a model that has been replicated throughout the country. A similar program focused on diabetes has also been very successful. In addition to programs such as these, many retail pharmacies are hiring those that live in these underserved communities where they understand the local culture and speak the language of the neighborhood.

Recent reports on how retail pharmacies are cutting corners regarding staffing the pharmacy counters has impacted much of the trust that retail pharmacies have gained through many of the partnering events that are described above. These media stories have created a challenging situation for retailers. First, the relationship with one's pharmacist is one of the leading indicators of trust and loyalty to a retail pharmacy. These stories have been based on complaints by pharmacists. In sharing their story, the pharmacists that are being interviewed are talking about the pressure that these staffing shortfalls have on both the pharmacists and the consumers that they are caring for. The pharmacists are pointing to the potential risk of medication errors that can occur with short staffing. In addition to the relationship with the pharmacist, customer service is another important factor in trust. Short staffing has been found to create longer lines and waiting at the pharmacy counter. Frustration associated with service delays creates lack of trust in the care that the consumer is receiving. Service and care often become inter-twined in the trust equation. We heard this earlier from Robert who shared that a dirty providers office impacted his trust of the doctor and from Gordie where the receptionist was sarcastic and rude to him impacting the trust of the care that he would receive. Trust has both intellectual and emotional attributes. (Knapp K, Ray M. et al. The Role of Community Pharmacies in Diabetes Care. July 2005)

One must ask the question as to how these changes in pharmacist practice and retail pharmacy impact the level of trust that a pharmacist has. A 2019 Gallup poll found that pharmacists are one of the most trusted professionals in the US. Honesty, ethical standards and accessibility lead the reason for this. The importance of this cannot be understated as most consumers have regular contact with a retail pharmacist whether it is to fill a prescription or to ask a question. There is a pharmacist at every corner. In fact, 90% of Americans lie within 2 miles of a pharmacy. They are the most accessible healthcare resource due to their location. Over the last few years there has been a slight decrease in trust of pharmacists. The reasons for this vary including the lack of consistency of the pharmacist/consumer relationship. As in other relationship based trusting relationships, length and depth of the relationship has a significant impact on levels of trust. It is not unusual for pharmacists to rotate from one store to another, especially in the larger retail chains. This has created challenges for pharmacists to create a relationship with those that they care for. In addition to the transient nature of the pharmacist in today's model, the customer experience has worsened, with often extended waiting times. Another area that creates trust challenges is in the case of a consumer being unable to access the medications that their providers prescribe. The retail pharmacist is often the individual that must tell the consumer that their drug is part of a prior authorization program or the price of a medication. In addition to these broader challenges, trust in retail pharmacists have been impacted due to the bad behavior of a few. In 1992, Robert Courtney, a retail pharmacist was found to dilute chemotherapy drugs of over 4200 patients. This case was covered by the national media and created a trust challenge for many pharmacists.

The relationship between pharmacists and consumers is not the only pivotal relationship that impacts trust within healthcare. The model of healthcare in the United States requires regular interaction between pharmacists and providers. Over the last 20 years, the relationship between the two healthcare professionals has been more adversarial than collegial. It is not unusual for pharmacists to reach out to prescribing providers either for clarification of the prescription, questions or recommendations regarding medication safety due to drug interactions or requesting changes in a prescription on behalf of a consumer in order to reduce consumer costs or for coverage reasons. Providers often feel disrupted, frustrated and in some cases angered by this type of interaction. It is perceived by the provider that prescribing is their role and that the pharmacist is interfering in the provider/ consumer relationship. Providers do not see this professional interaction as an integral part of medical care, in part due to the healthcare hierarchy and in part due to ego. Interactions such as these create a lack of trust and respect on both entities. Pharmacists we interviewed were divided in their experiences with physicians and other healthcare providers. There is a need for both organizations to find a path to collaboration. This will not only improve the relationship and confidence of the two professions but will also improve the trusting relationship with consumers and improve the outcomes of the care that is being given, as consumers often feel like they are placed in the middle of a professional argument.

Kai is a third- year pharmacy student. Kai shared her experience interacting with both prescribers and consumers. "I found it interesting that younger doctors were more open to my thoughts around medication management. They did not see my calls as second guessing them. This was not the case with many older doctors. Many of them talked down to me. One even told me never to call him again." "My interaction with patients has been different than my interactions with doctors. Patients are almost always appreciative of my thoughts and suggestions. Yes, they do ask me if I would talk to their doctors for them. They seemed to be concerned that their doctors will get mad at them if they discuss possible medication changes. Some seem to be afraid that they will be seen as not trusting their doctors. Most of the patients that I talk with think that all doctors and pharmacists work together and get along. "

The role of the pharmacist in the healthcare environment is changing. Today retail pharmacists are taking a greater role in the care of consumers, especially those with chronic conditions. Activities such as point in care testing, the giving of vaccines, and even under certain circumstances, prescribing medications are becoming more prevalent and are expected to grow. Pharmacists are also taking on greater responsibility within the healthcare team, rounding with other providers both in ambulatory and in- patient settings. It has become increasingly common to have a pharmacist as part of an oncology or ICU team supporting the medication decision making process. As these roles become more common, others within the healthcare environment will change their perception of the role of pharmacist. The pharmacist will no longer be perceived solely as a dispenser of medications. Their knowledge and expertise in medications will become more understood and respected. Respect and competence breed trust. I admit, I did not really understand the deep knowledge that pharmacists have regarding medications until I began working at Caremark and CVS Health. It took my about six months to realize that the pharmacists that I was working with were so much more knowledgeable about pharmacy. My trust in both the individuals that I worked with as well as the profession was elevated.

## Pharmacy Benefit Managers

Pharmacy benefit managers (PBMs) are the companies that have taken on the role of managing prescription drug benefits on behalf of employers, health plans and the government as a third -party administrator. The first PBM was founded in 1968. By the 1970s they began serving as an intermediary on behalf of payers. Since that time the role of the PBM has expanded. Their role varies depending on the individual contract and may include

- Developing and managing formularies or drug lists
- Negotiating drug costs through discounts and rebates
- Processing and paying prescription drug claims
- Negotiating the costs of dispensing medications with retail pharmacies
- Clinical programs to assure clinical appropriateness, safety and cost effectiveness

The primary role of the PBM is to manage the cost of medications on behalf of their clients. The role has become increasingly important as medication costs have risen significantly. The model that PBMs utilize has increasingly created questions across the industry. The basis for coverage decisions made by PBMs created more questions than answers. A 2019 study published in Health Affairs found that the studies used to create coverage policies were inconsistent across largest payers in the country. Only 15% of the of almost 5000 coverage decisions were similar. (Chambers et al., 2019) When asked how the studies were chosen, organizations answered that the most impactful and important studies were utilized. One may ask; if these are considered the most important studies why was there so little consistency? Was there no standardization? In most countries outside of the United States, decision- making and the use of science is standardized and transparent. Why not the United States? The answers given have not satisfied many. They have also created trust challenges. This lack of trust is not new. In 1998, the Department of Justice investigated the

PBM industry. The investigation was focused on the effectiveness of reducing prescription prices and whether they (PBMs)are focused on working on behalf of their clients. The questions regarding PBM practices have continued since that time.

One of the major areas of consternation and trust challenges focuses on rebates. Rebates are a tool that PBMs utilize during price negotiations with the pharmaceutical manufacturers. Studies have found that rebates have increased from $39.7 billion dollars in 2012 to $89.5 billion dollars in 2016. (The Commonwealth Fund, April 2019) PBMs state that a large portion of these rebates are passed on to employers and health plans. Research has found that this is often the case, but not always.

> Robin is a 39- year -old HR Benefits Director. Robin speaks about the rebate contract that her company has with the PBM that they contract with. "Rebates are necessary. We hate them but it helps us to keep premiums down for our employees. It is like finding a bucket full of quarters in the sofa. It is found money."

Regardless of Robins comments, payers are becoming increasingly distrustful of PBMs and the rebate model. When asked, employers and health plan executives feel that they are being "gamed." In addition to the issues associated with rebates, payers are concerned that there are additional dollars being paid to the PBMs outside of the rebates for activities and data and that revenues are not being shared with the payers although the money is based on activities associated with their employees and members. If trust is based on aligned goals, one needs to ask if the PBM goals are aligned with their clients or are PBMs using rebates and other payments they are receiving for their own purposes?

Lack of transparency and complexity of contracting is another area that payers say concern them. The opacity of contracting has created distrust. Many payers believe that the confusing contracts are a way for PBMs to muddle reimbursement mechanisms such as spread. Spread is when a PBM charges the payer one price and pays the retail pharmacy another price. PBMs answer to spread is that this differential helps to pay for those drugs where a PBM loses money. This revenue model is hard to audit and therefore creates some of the trust challenges. Payers have consistently requested greater transparency and simplification of contracting. To date, these demands have not been fulfilled. (Drettwan, J. Kjos A. An Ethical Analysis of Pharmacy Benefit Manager Practices. Pharmacy. June 2019. 7(2); 65. (doi.3390/pharmacy7020065)

## Employers Rate Trustworthiness and Satisfaction

| Vendor | Strongly Aligned | Very Trustworthy | Very Satisfied |
| --- | --- | --- | --- |
| Benefit Advisor/Consultant N=87 | 66% | 69% | 62% |
| Health Plan N=85 | 38% | 44% | 41% |
| PBM N=84 | 33% | 35% | 37% |
| SPM N=73* | 30% | 33% | 35% |

Responses on 1-7 Likert scale *number comprises respondents who report engaging with a SPM, including those who receive specialty pharmacy services from their PBM and those who contract with SPMs separately

Source: Stahl, Michael The price of filling a prescription: Independent pharmacies fight for survival Brooklyn Daily Eagle, May 20, 2019

The contractual relationship between the retail pharmacy and the PBM brings not only frustration and distrust from the payer, but it also creates distrust and anger in the retail pharmacy industry. FixRx, an advocacy group for retail pharmacies is fighting for the regulation of PBMs. The organization has stated that PBMs are creating a situation where retail pharmacies may become unviable due to the payment model that they are being forced into by the PBM industry. A survey done by FixRx found that "99 percent of those surveyed were concerned about abusive PBM practices." The PBM industry responded by saying that their responsibility is to their clients, the payers. Their clients are asking the PBMs to keep medications affordable. This means to aggressively negotiate payment terms with retail pharmacies on their clients (the payers) behalf. Over the last few years, both state and federal government has begun to discuss interceding in this disagreement. Regardless, there is little trust between the two organizations. (Stahl, Michael. The price of filling a prescription; Independent pharmacies fight for survival. Brooklyn Daily Eagle. May 20, 2019)

What about the consumer? How do PBM actions impact them? Is it the role of the PBM to assure that the consumer is not negatively impacted by their actions? The fiduciary relationship does not include the consumer and therefore it is not the responsibility of the PBM to consider the consumer as the client. Decisions that PBMs make have a direct impact on consumers. These decisions have both a clinical and financial impact. The rebates that are collected from manufacturers do not lower the cost of the medication for a consumer. In fact, the rebate model often increases the gross cost of the medication and that is what the consumers price is based on. What does this mean, consumers pay more due to the rebate model? What do consumers think about PBMs? As we interviewed consumers regarding their feelings about PBMs we heard:

1. Consumers do not really understand the PBM model. They do know that they have a drug card that is supposed to help them pay for their medicines. They know that the cost of their medicines is going up. They do not know who to blame, so they blame everyone.

2. They know that they often are unable to get the drug that their doctor has prescribed for them due to rules that are made by the PBM or health insurance company. They trust their provider to give them the correct drug. They do not trust those organizations that create a barrier to that care

3. The service that consumers receive when they reach out to the PBM is most often unsatisfactory. They are unable to get answers to the questions that they have and frequently do not get the outcome they are hoping for.

Overall, consumers have low levels of trust in the PBM industry. It is an industry that they do not understand. In addition, the recent increased opportunity to use drug cards and programs such as GoodRx, outside of their PBM drug benefit have become more prevalent. Their experience is that they can get some of their medications at prices considerably lower than they can through their drug benefit. These drug cards do not create the same barriers that their PBM does.

Pharmacy services are a large and diverse group of organizations. How they are perceived varies as does the trust level of each of the organizations. The convoluted methods used in determining price across these services has created animosity and a lack of trust both within this part of the industry as well as for those that are effected. This group of organizations are a good example of how trust can be impacted by the misalignment of goals and a lack of transparency within each organization as well as across organizations.

## Technology and Trust

Technology is all around us. Over the last decade technology has become commonplace within our lives. We communicate through it, shop through it, clean our houses using it.

- 96% of Americans have cell phones with 81% of them being smartphones (Pew Research)
- 74% of Americans own a computer (Statistica)
- $269 billion dollars were spent via ecommerce in 2019. This was prior to the pandemic. (Statistica)

In addition to the use of technology in our daily lives, technology is taking an ever -increasing role in health and healthcare.

- 21% of consumers are using health apps and wearable trackers. (Pew)

- 72% of consumers use the internet to research health information. (Becker's Hospital Review)
- 15% of all surgeries include some type of robot assisted procedures. (Sheetz K. Claflin J. et al. Trends in the Adoption of Robotic Surgery for Common Surgical Procedures. JAMA. Jan. 10,2020; 3(1))
- Healthcare data is growing at a 36% annualized rate with as much as 30% of the worlds stored data being generated by the healthcare industry. (Huesch M. Mosher T. Using it or Losing It? NEJM May 4, 2017.)

We need to start by defining what we mean by health and healthcare technology. The definition varies depending on whom you ask. The World Health Organization defines technology as "the application of organized knowledge and skills in the form of devices drugs, medical and surgical equipment and systems to address a medical problem." Many include data and analytics within the definition and others do not. For our purposes, we will utilize a broad definition of health and medical technology. Regardless of how you define health and healthcare technology, we all agree it is used by all the stakeholders across the healthcare environment.

Why has technology become so important in the healthcare environment? The goal of technology is to increase effectiveness, efficiency, safety and convenience in order to identify healthcare problems earlier, treat disease in a less invasive manner and at times to reduce costs. Technology has become a change agent and led to the democratization in some areas of healthcare due to the equalizing of available knowledge. In order to achieve these goals, it is important that potential utilizers of technology trust it.

When discussing technology and trust within the healthcare environment one must talk about the trust that individuals or organizations have in the technology itself as well as how technology has impacted trust between individuals within healthcare. Let's start discussing trust of technology. A 2019 Edelman trust barometer found several interesting factoids regarding technology and trust including:

1.  Technology as an industry has had high levels of trust.
2.  We are going through a "techlash." This is defined by Oxford Dictionary as "strong and widespread negative reaction" to technology. This backlash is partly due to the growing power and influence that large technology companies have. There is fear as to how this power is being utilized.
3.  Data privacy and power over the consumers information are major drivers of this lack of trust and techlash.

Trust in technology is multi-dimensional and constantly evolving. The trust in this environment has been found to be directly related to the experience that an individual has while using the technology. Abbas and his co-authors found a cadre of variables that can impact the trust of technology. In most cases, trust has also been found to increase as the technology is used more and the individual becomes more comfortable with it. Think of it as building a relationship with the technology. This is especially true with healthcare providers use of technology. One good example of this can be found in the use of robotic technology used during surgery. In 2012 robotics were only used 1.8% of the time. By 2018 that percentage has risen to over 15%. Not all providers are trusting of the technology. There are a number of reasons for this lack of trust by providers. One common reason for issues associated with distrust have to do with a previous bad experience with technology.

> Sidney is an OB-Gyn (obstetrics and gynecology) doctor. He shared with us his lack of trust in technology. "I have done hundreds of hysterectomies in my career. Our group decided to begin offering robotic assisted laparoscopy for hysterectomies. I found it was taking almost twice as long and had a whole new set of risks associated with it. I just did not trust this method. Too much could go wrong"

I went on to ask him whether any of his patients had experienced complications. His answer was yes, twice. After that he went back to the more traditional methods of surgery. "After all my years of training, I trust my hands more than I do this other machinery."

In some cases, it is less about actual trust and more about the competition they feel with technology. A 2019 article from The Brookings Institute talked about the potential for robots to replace doctors. There are instances in healthcare where the technology has shown equal or better quality of care than the provider. A 2017 MIT study showed this when it compared radiologists reviewing mammograms to artificial intelligence reviewing the same radiologic studies. (Kocher et al, 2019)

| Trust Facilitators | Trust Barriers |
| --- | --- |
| Compatibility | Privacy and security |
| Security | Lack of efficiency |
| Reliability | Cost |
| Functionality | Quality |
| Perceived Usefulness | Perceived risk of use |
| Training and technical support | Complexity |
| Usability | Poor training and support |

Source: Abbas, 2018

Often it is not the technology itself that providers do not trust, it is the impact of the technology that they feel can negatively impact trust. Earlier In the book we met Mary Felipe and Chris her husband. Both are primary care providers. During our conversation we asked them about technology. Very quickly Chris spoke up" Technology is important, but it can also be very disruptive. The electronic medical record (EMR)we use is supposed to help with documentation and decision support. That may be the case. Unfortunately, it impacts how I interact with my patients. If I am typing into the EMR, I am not paying attention to my patient, I am not looking them in the eye, and I am missing body language. The EMR is a barrier to relationships and that impacts the trust that my patients have in me."

It is not just providers that are utilizing technology for health and healthcare purposes. One in five adults are following their own metrics for things such as blood pressure, blood sugar, heart rate or number of steps taken. Although more consumers are utilizing technology, more than 50% of consumers have voiced their skepticism about whether there are benefits. In addition to self -monitoring tools, consumers are exposed to technologies such as patient portals, electronic medical records and technologies to support telehealth.

Recently, we have seen a significant increase in the use of virtual technology- based visits between consumers and their providers. Adoption of this type of care has been rising. Physician adoption in 2019 was 28% and consumer adoption was up 30% over the previous year. The COVID pandemic of 2020 changed that. Consumers were unable to see providers in a face-to-face situation. Over a three- month period, 71% of consumers had considered telemedicine. A further study found that 83% of consumers expect to continue to use telehealth in the future. An article in the July 14, 2020 JAMA by Dr. Marcin Chwistek, talks about a woman that prior to starting a telemedicine visit with her physician asks him "Are you wearing your white coat?" The patient goes on to say that this is how she needs to imagine him. Although the question seems to be a simple one, it teaches us an important lesson about technology. Technology can be an efficient and sometimes effective tool. It is not the most effective relationship building tool. Yes, newer technologies that allow us to see each other faces is helpful, it is not as effective in conveying and sharing emotions and not effective in allowing for a handshake or touch. Personal contact and all that it brings to the relationship is lost when utilizing technology.

Providers trust in health technology differs from consumers trust in technology. Providers base trust on the trustworthiness of the system as well as their comfort in the use of the technology. Consumers trust in technology utilized by their providers is tied to their trust in their provider. Consumers are often concerned that their providers are not proficient in the use of technology. Their concern is based on fear of injury. In addition to the concern over use of the technology itself, trust is also tied to what they believe that their providers and others will do with the information that is gathered from the technology. In fact, the leading barriers to trusting technology for consumers is concerns over privacy and security. Many of those surveyed stated that they withheld information due to their lack of trust. (Shaw G. 2017).

There is a common belief that the use of technology and the trust in that technology is associated with the age of the consumer. This is only partially true. Age does not have as significant an impact as many believe. Seniors are willing to use technology. Technology has played a significant role in many individuals work life. As consumers age into Medicare and transition into retirement, these individuals are comfortable utilizing and trusting in technologies. Many other seniors are using technology such as smartphones, tablets or computers to communicate with family members in other cities.

A Pew Survey released September16, 2020 has shown that a majority of Americans (1213 individuals over the age of 18 were surveyed) support the sharing of medical information between those that are caring for them. In addition, they want greater access to their own data. Those that were older were slightly less interested. The greatest concern that they had was in privacy. They articulated a need for federal health data protections. (Moscovitch Ben. Americans Want Federal Government to Make Sharing Electronic Health Data Easier. Pew Research. September 20, 2020)

Pew Research Center and Accenture have been following technology trends in the senior market for several years. Both organizations have seen increasing use of technology in this population. Both organizations found that seniors show an increasing comfort in using technology.

---

Pew Research Centers' survey on the Internet and American Life Project found that:

- 40% of seniors own and use a smart phone,
- over 69% use the internet regularly.
- Over 30% own a tablet and use social media,
- 58% use the internet to find healthcare information and
- 43% use Facebook to research information.
- 60% of seniors are willing to wear health monitoring devices to track their health.

---

Seniors and Healthcare Technology

- 83% feel that they should have full access to their electronic health records
- 68% feel that it is important to request their prescriptions electronically
- 62% use the internet to find health information
- 62% believe it is important to be able to book appointments electronically
- 53% feel it is important to email with their providers
- 66% want technology to access care from home

Accenture 2015

---

Seniors trust in technology is mediated by many of the same factors as consumers of other ages. These factors include privacy of information, credibility of the company, and reliability. Areas where seniors differ than younger consumers are the significant impact on trust that technical difficulties caused by key size, font size, and the complexity and frustration of comprehending directions. One other area that has a significant impact on trust who suggests the use of the technology. Older consumers trust technology suggested by their doctors and their friends. An interesting issue that needs to be pointed out is the fact that family carries less credibility than friends regarding technology use for healthcare. We found this to be the case with two individuals that we interviewed

> Duffy is a 78-year-old gentleman that lives alone after the death of his wife. Duffy explained that his children wanted him to have a home safety unit in case he was to fall. Duffy did not want the unit in his house as he felt that he was being spied on by his children. "My kids are always asking me what I am doing and if I am ok. I feel like this box thing that they want to put in my house, will tell them how many beers I am drinking and what I am eating."

> Isabella is a 69-year-old woman that has diabetes and heart disease. She is on eight medications.
> She was given an automated pill container that organizes her medicines. Isabella shared her frustration over the use of the pill container. "I ran over the container with my car. I don't like having a pill box yell at me. I got so frustrated, I had to destroy it. Only after my doctor explained to me the importance of my medicines, did I agree to try again."

Technology has been a two -edged sword in healthcare. There are those that believe that technology and the digitalization of healthcare has impacted trust. Some say that technology has brought greater trust through the increased access for those that would not otherwise have access and creating an efficient means of communication between individuals making information available often in a timely and easy manner. Others feel that trust has been significantly bruised due to overpromising on results, not addressing the privacy concerns or replacing important relationships that are foundational to the trust in the system. Technology cannot hug you when you are frightened or in pain. If we are to increase the integration of technology into our health solutions, we will have to be focused on doing so in an aligned and transparent manner.

## The Media

> Knowledge is Power
> Thomas Jefferson

Media is a stakeholder that rarely comes to mind when talking about the players and influencers within the healthcare environment. The reality is that media has a significant impact on all the stakeholders within the healthcare environment as it lays a foundation for perceptions that can impact trust and its impact can be almost instantaneous. There are few that were alive in 1963 that do not remember Walter Cronkite crying on national television as he shared the news of President John F Kennedy's death. During that time, he was considered by many to be the most trusted man in America.

### THE DEFINITION OF MEDIA

Oxford dictionary defines the term media as a "means of mass communication." The problem is that not everyone agrees as to what constitutes media. For many years the main format of media was the written word. The era of the written word as the main disseminator of information began with the printing press. Many have stated that the printing press is one of the inventions that has had the greatest impact on civilization. The printing press allowed for information to be shared more broadly and more quickly. The use of the printing press led to the first newspaper being started in 1704. The press as a conduit to trusted information was considered so important during these early periods of American history that it was memorialized in the First Amendment of the Bill of Rights.

Newspapers and print remained the major form of media until the 1920s. Like newspapers, radio played an important role in the distribution of information. NBC and CBS radio created both news and entertainment features that were broadcast on a regular basis. Franklin Roosevelt as president utilized the radio as an influencing tool. Eight days after being inaugurated as President of the United States, Roosevelt made a radio speech trying to convince the public that the economy was stable. His regular radio "fireside chats" created a long and trusting relationship between himself and the country.

Although newspapers and radio remained important tools, television broke into the media world in the 1950s. Early television journalists such as Edward R. Morrow became important and influential information conduits. Increasingly television brought both news and entertainment to the masses. During this period, there were three major networks: NBC, ABC and CBS. We watched the nightly news to find out what was happening in the world. Trust at that time for the media was high. During this time, the news was informational with little editorial or entertainment aspect to it. Those of us alive at the time of the President John F. Kennedy assassination will not forget Walter Cronkite tearing up on national television. His public vulnerability brought trust to an even higher level of trust than he already had with the public. The world watched in 1969 when Neil Armstrong and Buss Aldrin made history by beeing the first individuals to step foot on the moon. It was during President Nixon's time that the terms "the press" and "mainstream media" were first used. The 1980s saw several momentous changes to the news and media world that would forever alter the industry and the public's trust in the information that was disseminated. First, 1980 brought CNN and the advent of the 24 hours a day news. This required programming and stations that had previously been focused on information to broaden their programming. News began to be informational intertwined with entertainment. The second major change was the increased use of data that was being collected by media outlets. The data being collected was now being used to target market and target message. This created siloed information presented to subpopulations of individuals in order to influence both their beliefs and actions. A final major change then took place in the 1990s with the public facing use of the internet. Although the internet began within the military in the 1960s, it did not go "mainstream" until the 1990s. This transition began the world of the "commercial internet". Since that time, we have seen a massive increase in consumers use of the internet and broadening in how they use it. In addition to information seeking, the internet has been used as a communication conduit through social media. The evolution of the internet has impacted numerous aspects of our lives. It has now created a world of the "last five minutes" in the world of information flow. The data and demographic micro-segmentation that began in the 1980s was hyper-powered via utilization of the internet. There is a common belief that these changes created a forty-year downward trend of trust across all forms of media.

The last fifteen years has once again brought significant changes to the media ecosystem. Social media has increased while more traditional forms of media such as newspapers, periodicals, news shows on both radio and traditional television has decreased. More sophisticated use of data has created social media algorithms that further the use of micro-messaging. In addition, social media has created an environmental rise in what is often called "fake news." The term fake news is used for information that is untrue but presented as truthful. Like other factors we see, fake news has created a cloud of mistrust for all information. Lines between content, opinion and commerce have become so blurred that little is trusted. (Aspen Institute 2019)

There are a growing number of organizations that are offering information via the internet and social media. We need to ask whether fake news really has an impact on consumers, organizations and society.

There are two immediate concerns regarding fake news, first is the fact that it is often difficult to detect the difference between fake news and news that has been substantiated by trusted sources. The second concern is that all information and news is increasingly doubted because of the lack of clear differentiation between fake news and substantiated information. In order to gain or retain trust, news providers need to be transparent regarding the source of information, and when possible associate themselves with trusted individuals or organizations.

As information has become more available, the impact of media regardless of source has intensified. This impact focuses on four areas including: acquisition, triggering, altering and reinforcing. The unfortunate part of this is that although the information that is being shared is trusted by many of those receiving it, the information is not always correct. (Borah, P. 2016)

---

Media Effects

1. Acquiring- a person obtains information or ideas that they did not have prior to the exposure
2. Triggering-the media influences a person by activating something that already existed
3. Altering-the media influences a person to change something that they already had
4. Reinforcing- the media influences a person by making something in the person more difficult to change

The Encyclopedia of Political Communication 2016

---

## THE MEDIA AND ITS IMPACT ON HEALTHCARE

Media plays a prominent role in healthcare for both consumers and providers. Media has created the democratization of healthcare by allowing society a wide understanding of healthcare information, attributes and interactions. 69% of U.S. adults that say that they learn about doctors, medical specialties and how healthcare works through the news media. (Pew) Unfortunately, a significant portion of the information is incorrect. This was true in the 1960s and continues to be true today. Americans are inundated with news. The average American hears approximately 100,000 words daily through some form of media. These words have an impact on what we think and who we trust. This ecosystem of information has caused a great deal of confusion. As humans, confusion often leads to mistrust. As mass media has increasingly played a role in health and healthcare information it is important to look at how it is perceived by those that are receiving these messages and its impact on our healthcare system. More than 50% of Americans (59%) stated that they are distrustful of the information that is reported. This study focuses mainly on newspapers, television and radio and does not take social media into consideration. (Brenan M. Americans Trust in Mass Media Edges Down to 41%. Politics, September 26, 2019) The Edelman Trust Barometer found that media has a significant impact on trust in healthcare. It does not matter whether the media conduit providing this information is radio, television, periodicals or newspapers or social media.

Television and movies have played a significant role in impacting trust in healthcare. It has both confused and clarified healthcare issues and the roles that each stakeholder plays within the environment. I grew up in the 1960s watching medical based television shows. Most of these shows ended with a happy ending. I thought all physician's practices were like Dr Marcus Welby with his nurse Juanita and his medical partner Dr Steven Kiley. You never saw medical errors, care denials or high medical bills. I do not know about you, but there is little truth to that story. Each generation has their television shows about medicine. Grey's Anatomy, Marcus Welby, ER, or House. During the year of 2000-2001 television did not have a single positive reference to healthcare. In 2002, Turow and his fellow authors found that in a review of weekly medical television, every show had a subplot focused on a public policy issue. Again, this is not reality. It is not just television. John Q, a popular movie that was released in 2002, was focused on a character played by Denzel Washington, who was fighting with his health insurance carrier to pay for his son's heart transplant. This movie created the belief that all insurance companies were evil and not to be trusted.

It is not just television shows or movies that carry these messages, they are also transmitted by news outlets, both written and visual. Media rarely talks about the "good news stories" in healthcare. Good news does not sell or help ratings, sensationalism does. Therefore, much of what the consumer sees is sensationalized, whether it is true or not. What we hear about is nursing home deaths, pharmacists diluting cancer medications, pharmaceutical companies raising medication prices and health plans withholding care. One study found that over a twelve year period there were twenty-six hundred news stories that were found to include information that was incorrect regarding benefits, harms and costs of the healthcare interventions discussed. These are the kind of stories that create distrust in the system. (Arora, 2020)

In addition to medical treatments and breakthroughs, the media often reports on stories that focus on how healthcare organizations are paid or the misdeeds of one organization or another. An example of this is Heather Bresch, the CEO of or Mylan. Over a seven -year period the cost of the EpiPen increased from $103.50 to $608.61. Bresch was called to testify in front of Congress regarding this significant cost increase. This controversy made all the news outlets and created outrage. Another example of this was the news coverage regarding Theranos. The healthcare technology company was formed in 2003 and was valued at $200 billion dollars in 2014. The founder Elizabeth Holmes was regarded as a genius and was frequently interviewed in the press. In 2015, John Carreyrou, a writer for the Wall Street Journal received a tip and exposed the company as a scam. In 2018, the company ceased operations after being sanctioned by CMS and sued by organizations such as Walgreens. In addition, both Elizabeth Holmes and Ramesh (Sunny) Balwani were charged with fraud by the SEC. This story has been told numerous times through the written and other forms of media through articles, books, movies and TV News segments. The Theranos story has led to a further reduction of trust. Both of these ethically challenged organizations led to the average consumer and health care providers distrusting both. In several of our interviews we found that the interviewees believe that the pharmaceutical manufacturers as a whole overcharge and are disreputable.

As media modalities evolve, the opportunities and challenges for communication and interaction broaden. Over the last fifteen years social media as an additional means of disseminating health information has increased. Social media and trust can positively impact a consumer's ability for self -trust regarding health and healthcare. This form of media has brought with it new levels of just in time information as well the ability to micro focus information at an individual level. Consumers are using social media for a myriad of purposes including gathering information and communicating with others. The dissemination of facts and information are important to decision making in healthcare. A 2011 study stated that 40% of those surveyed stated that social media is very likely or likely to impact their future healthcare decisions. The Health Research Institute of pwc found that 42% of consumers are using social media to find physicians, hospitals and treatment options. They also found that over 25% have posted information regarding their own health status and 20% have reached out to join a health- related community group.

Do online health seekers trust social media? A study commissioned by Weber Shandwick and KRC Research found that Americans who use social media for health information have concerns about incorrect or misleading information. This has created trust issues both in social media as an information source but also for those that believe in social media it can impact lack of trust in healthcare.

Over the last few years, there has been an increase in control by unknown sources in social media. This has created concerns over both the validity of the information as well as issues associated with data and privacy. (Webershadwick.com November 13, 2018) (The Great American Search for Healthcare Information Healthcare Social Media. April 3, 2020) (Smailhodzic E. Hooijsma W. et al. Social Media Use in Healthcare: A systemic review of effects on patients and their relationship with healthcare professionals. BMC Health Services Research. 2016; 16(1); 442)

The status of facts is not what it used to be. It is often inconsistent, biased, or 'fake'" We define fake or false information as that without supporting scientific evidence. This can be especially true of information shared via social media. If the facts are incorrect, it may lead to a media effect that can be deleterious to the consumer, including poor outcomes or complete loss of trust in all that they read, hear and see

Confusing and conflicting information can be just as damaging to trust as false or incorrect information. It is often hard for consumers to distinguish what information is correct and which is false. Is caffeine good for you or not? Can I eat eggs every morning or will it raise my cholesterol? Do hormone medications after menopause raise my risk of breast cancer or heart disease? A recent study found that 80% of those with a chronic condition received conflicting information between their doctor, the media, and the internet. This creates a situation of lack of trust.

> Julie, when asked whether she trusts the media when it comes to health and healthcare issues stated" I don't know who to trust and when you do not know who to trust, you trust no one."

This loss of trust can also make health and healthcare decision making much more difficult. Facts are no longer believed to be "right and true." The concern "science versus science fiction" negates the positive impact of social media as a health tool. (Merchant)

Where do consumers turn when they are confused or need information? When they are unsure, they often turn to those that they trust. Our survey shows that consumers look to doctors, hospital and pharmacists to get the healthcare information that they most trust. Only 20 % saying they found trusted information online

As our research stated, a provider, such as the pediatrician, Dr Judy that we met earlier is often relied upon for information. Dr Judy's patient came to her with asthma information that was found on the internet. Dr Judy was able to help her patient to understand what was correct and where to seek out information in the future. In other cases, consumers turn to friends and family. Although these individuals are often trusted, they may or may not know any more than other than the consumer. Trust does not always protect the consumer from misinformation.

The survey results below from, *The Great American Search for Healthcare Information*, was conducted among 1,700 Americans 18 years of age and older. It was commissioned by global communications and marketing services firm Weber Shandwick in partnership with KRC Research and published in November of 2018.

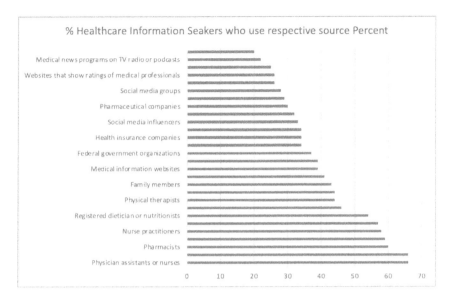

**% Healthcare Information Seakers who use respective source Percent**

Medical news programs on TV radio or podcasts
Websites that show ratings of medical professionals
Social media groups
Pharmaceutical companies
Social media influencers
Health insurance companies
Federal government organizations
Medical information websites
Family members
Physical therapists
Registered dietician or nutritionists
Nurse practitioners
Pharmacists
Physician assistants or nurses

0   10   20   30   40   50   60   70

**Sources used by 50 or more healthcare information seekers**
**Source:(Adapted from the Weber Shandwick and KRC https://www.prnnewswrie.com)**

In addition to their healthcare providers, consumers often look to other consumers for help. Social media is one way that is utilized by consumers to communicate with others that are challenged with similar health issues. Organizations such as Patients Like Me or other social media based "smart health communities" exist so that consumers can feel a sense of community and interact with others having similar experiences. Dr Dhar, the Chief Health Informatics Officer at Deloitte found that these virtual communities act in similar ways to actual communities. (Dhar, 2019) He identified areas in which these communities impact the health of the consumers that engage including:

1. Foster a sense of community
2. Utilize health data and behavioral science
3. Create and improve health ecosystems
4. Reduce isolation and loneliness
5. Drive the ability of a consumer to engage in their own care
6. Improve health outcomes

Although many of these 'communities' and interactions have positive impact, others have been shown to create further confusion and dissemination of biased or incorrect information. Many of these interactions are solely peer moderated. This creates the opportunity for the sharing of incorrect information.

Media does not only impact healthcare consumers, but it also impacts healthcare providers. Providers, like consumers, utilize a variety of media types depending on what they are trying to achieve. Television and news have an impact on providers perceptions, behaviors and levels of trust.

> Dr. Daria is a 56- year -old physician. We asked her about her feelings when she reads or hears about healthcare issues such as Theranos or Mylan. "Things that negatively impact patients makes me angry. Companies such as these (Theranos and Mylan), lead me to distrust organizations. They are all out to make money and not to help people. I hate listening to the news."

The most utilized form of media that providers utilize is the medical journal. Providers rely on journals and other healthcare focused media to help stay up to date and aware of new and changing healthcare trends. A report from the Journal of American Medical Library Association found that over 7000 articles are published monthly in primary care journals alone. A 2015 Doximity study found that.

- 98% of physicians report that reading medical literature is important
- 44% state that they spend at least 1-2 hours a week reading news online, while 22% state they spend 3-4 hours a week reading medical news online.

What happens when the information in those journals is found to be misleading? It is not just the popular press that offers incorrect information. Over the last few years there has been increasing concern from providers about the reliability of the information that they receive from journals and other sources. Recent stories have contained poor research, the information conveyed is exaggerated or withheld, and. in a few instances, lies about findings.

Providers do not just rely on medical journals and periodicals as tools. They also utilize social media. There are numerous social media tools that have been created specifically for healthcare providers including social networking platforms, blogs, media sharing sites and most recently provider-patient virtual care sites. The most common internet and social media sites utilized by providers is focused on new and existing scientific information. New scientific evidence that is published through traditional methods (written journals) can take over a year whereas social media can get the information out in a very short period. Although social media can positively impact new and important scientific information, it also can disseminate information that can be incorrect or misleading. A 2019 article found that the quality and reliability of the information found on social media is the biggest drawback of this media format. The more traditional means of dissemination such as peer reviewed journals have safety hurdles in place in order to decrease misinformation or fake news. These safety hurdles such as peer review are not utilized in most social media or alternative forms of information dissemination. Funding sources for social media sites vary. Funding can have a significant impact on what is displayed and the level of trust from providers. Hidden agendas and conflicts of interest can be difficult to access in social media.

In addition to funding, privacy issues associated with social media are often a concern to providers. Some of the social media sites have addressed these privacy concerns by creating Health Insurance

Portability and Accountability Act (HIPAA) compliant sites. These types of actions have gone a long way in addressing the trust issues that providers have articulated.

It does not matter the stakeholder or the media type, information is trusted when the sharing party is a trusted individual or organization. Who shares the information has a significant impact on whether individuals trust this information. This is regardless of the original source of the information. The study found that people who see media-based information will trust it more if it is sent by someone, they trust regardless of the media source. It goes on to show that they are likely to share that post or article if it was sent by a credible source. "The sharers act as unofficial ambassadors for the brand, and sharers credibility can influence readers opinions about the reporting source." (Who Shared it; How Americans Decide what News to Trust on Social Media. March 20, 2017). It is clear, trust begets trust.

## Who Shares the Information Matters

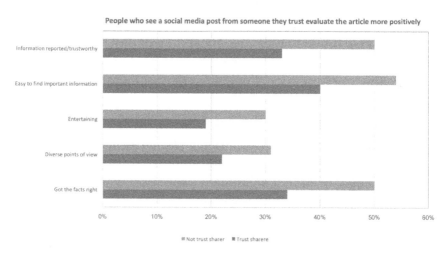

People who see a social media post from someone they trust evaluate the article more positively

Source: Media Insight Project

## The Government's Impact on Trust

> Lorraine is a 29- year- old teacher. When asked about her level of trust of the United States Government Lorraine laughed and said, "If you want something to take twice as long, cost twice as much and still not work, ask the government."

Trust in the American government was at 75% in 1964. Most of the country believed that the federal government would do the right thing. Unfortunately, this high level of trust has shown a consistent downward trend since that time. A portion of this distrust originates from the increasing level of political polarization that has occurred over the last forty years. Beginning in the late 1970s individuals such as Newt Gingrich began to speak about the competitive nature of the human. He compared it to the animal world where aggressiveness is natural and is the only way to survive. This has led to a large group of government officials "raising hell, stopped being so nice and believe that politics and the government it produces is a war for power. The era of conversation and compromise was ending" (Coppins, 2018). A second factor that has impacted trust in Washington is the lack of relationships that exist both within a party and especially across party lines. Until the late 1980s most congressmen and senators lived a large portion of their lives in Washington DC and not in the state that they were representing. It was difficult to use hate speech against someone with whom you went to PTA meetings or worshiped with. Socializing builds relationships which in turn builds trust. This lack of trust between governmental officials is contagious and has been passed on to the public. It has been well documented how elected officials of different parties who would argue during the day but have respectful personal relationships; individuals such as President Ronald Reagan and House Speaker Tip O'Neill, Senators John Kerry and John McCain and Senators Orin Hatch and Ted Kennedy. A quote by Orin Hatch of his relationship with Ted Kennedy exemplifies how these relationships worked; "I have to say that we became very dear friends. That doesn't mean we didn't fight each other. We fought like tooth and tongue but afterward, we'd put our arms around each other and laugh about it. We respected each other and trusted each other" (Panetta, 2018). Unfortunately, these types of relationships are rarely found today. Individuals sit across the aisle from one another and glare. There are rarely examples of bipartisan agreement. This creates an atmosphere of 'blood games.' This posturing creates a partisan feeling across the country leading to distrust of the 'other party' in Washington and the 'other party' in one's neighborhood or family.

> Filipe is a 28-year-old male. During our interview Filipe was very direct in his answer about his lack of trust in the government. "Politicians forget that their role is to do the right thing for the country. I do not believe that this is what is happening. Both federal and state politicians are worse than my twin three- year- old's. They talk at each other, have temper tantrums and threaten to take their ball and go home. This is not adult behavior that anyone in their right mind would trust."

A survey done by Georgetown University and NYU researchers found that consumers trust Amazon more than they trust the government. A 2019 study by the Commonwealth Fund and the Harvard T.H. Chan School of Public Health that questioned 2005 individuals over the age of 18 found that 69% of Americans have a negative, distrustful view of the government. They believe that things run by the United States government do not run well. Those that we interviewed are similar in their lack of trust. The reasons for this lack of confidence varies with some believing that the government does too much, while others believe the government does too little. Still others feel that the government performs its functions poorly. The most frequent response accused the leaders of focusing on remaining in office, maintaining their personal and party power and their overall lack of transparency. Regardless of the reasoning, few trusted that the government could successfully oversee issues that were important to them.

## The government as a healthcare payer

Healthcare has been a "kitchen table" issue for approximately forty years. A 2019 Survey done by Real Clear Opinion Research showed that healthcare is the leading issue for 36% of Americans. Those surveyed stated that the healthcare system needed improvement with only 4% stating that healthcare did not need any changes at this time. (Cannon, C. Medicare For All Support is High...But it's Complicated. May 15, 2019. RealClearPolitics. Com)

Top Issue Facing Americans Today

1. Healthcare 36%
2. Economy 26%
3. Immigration 15%
4. Education 11%
5. Environment 11%
6. Foreign Policy 3%

Real Clear Opinion Research May 2019

Many Americans see healthcare as the most pressing issue in their life. In conjunction with this belief, over 65% of Americans believe that the government has a significant role in improving the healthcare system. At the same time, less than 50% trust the government to take care of their health. over 65% of Americans believe that the government has a role in improving our healthcare system. (Pew Research Center, Americans View of Government: Low Trust but Some Positive Performance Ratings. September 14, 2020) This contradiction in beliefs is not the only one that we have identified. Many of those that shared their distrust of the government and their ability to perform also articulated their positive view of Medicare.

So how do we unwind these issues to make some sense of these conflicting paradoxical beliefs? The United States government's role in healthcare is one of the most debated topics in the United States. This is not a new subject. This debate goes back to the 1960s as the Government was working through the issues surrounding the passage of the Medicare Act of 1965 which established Medicare and Medicaid. (McPhillips Deidre. Majority of Americans Don't Trust Government with their Health. U.S. News and World Report. March 26, 2020) Medicare which covers all consumers over the age of 65 is very popular. While there is a significant opposition to the increased role by the U.S. government in healthcare, many consumers forget that Medicare is a government program. A 2014 poll found 41% of consumers felt that "making sure all Americans have healthcare coverage is a responsibility of the Federal government". A portion of those that did not feel that the government has a role in healthcare do so because of their belief in "small government" while other disagree with the statement due to their lack of trust in the government as a whole. To a large degree, this belief is due to lack of trust in the government. In 1964 78% of consumers trusted the federal government. Since that time the number of those that trust the government has decreased significantly. By 2020 that number was only at 20% according to Pew Research Center. (Dalen, J. Waterbrook K, Alpert J. Why do so Many Americans Oppose the Affordable Care Act? The American Journal of Medicine. 128(8). August 2015; 807-810). A 2020 Pew survey found that 19% of those surveyed felt that the government was doing a good job in ensuring safe medicine and 14% that the federal government was doing a good job in ensuring access to healthcare and 11% was doing an effective job in handling threats to public health. Only 20% stated that they trust the Federal government to "do the right thing." This becomes especially important at times of national healthcare challenges such as the COVID 19 pandemic of 2020. This debate continues.

When asked why consumers don't trust the government, many reasons are given. For young people, the lack of trust stems from basic philosophical differences, whereas for others it may be due to the partisan nature of our country today and for others it may be past direct or historical actions of the government. Events such as the Tuskegee Study in which members of the Black community were untreated for syphillis, the forced sterilizations of those that were considered "feeble minded" without their consent in the 1920s and a deceptive 1989 CDC study in which members of the Black and Hispanic community were given an experimental measles vaccine have created significant barriers to trust both inside and outside of the minority community. (Singleton, 2019)

In communities of color trust in healthcare under the auspices of the government was never regained.

---

The Federal Government Actions regarding Health and Healthcare

- 19% very good rating in ensuring safe medicine
- 14% very good rating in ensuring access to healthcare
- 11% very good rating in effectively handling threats to public health

Pew Research Center Aug. 2020

---

It is not only individual consumers that distrust the American government, most health insurers, health systems, healthcare service organizations and providers also distrust the government on issues surrounding healthcare. Like consumers, the reasons for this distrust of the government vary. Some of the healthcare leaders we spoke to talked about the fact that the United States is one of the few countries that politicizes health and healthcare issues.

Saria is the COO of a National Home Health Company. She shared that "since President Clinton, healthcare has become the tip of the sword. Issues surrounding healthcare are pawns in a bloody battle that has little to do with America and Americans. I don't trust most government employees to do what is right. That is not their focus."

We heard three common themes from Healthcare leaders regarding their lack of trust in the government regarding their interactions with the healthcare industry. The first focused on the fact that Government does not have a personal "face." The government is large and complex therefore there is no one person to consult on the matter. The second issue has to do with past experiences and frustrations in dealing with the government. These challenges create low expectations and increase the lack of trust. The third subject focuses on those in the government lacking the knowledge of how the industry works. This lack of knowledge creates situations during which while trying to solve one problem the government creates three new problems and increases the burden placed on the healthcare industry. (Lee et al)

Kelly is the CEO of a 6 -hospital system. In speaking with Kelly, he shared an example of the government mandating cost transparency by hospitals. "Cost transparency sounds good as a sound bite. The problem is that no one in the government thought to come and speak with us. They have no idea all the challenges that are associated with making this happen. The cost to creating a cost transparent system will be greater than the savings that the government is hoping to achieve."

Regardless of whether one believes that the government should have a significant role in healthcare; everyone would agree that the U.S. government does have an impact on the healthcare system, whether as the largest payer in the United States, the overseer of many impactful organizations associated with the countries health and healthcare, or as the creator of policy and law that directly or indirectly affects the healthcare system. The government is front and center in the healthcare environment.

## The Government as a Payer

Today the United States government is the largest single payor of healthcare in the United States through programs that it sponsors such as Medicare, Medicaid, State Children's Health Insurance (SCHIP), the Department of Defense and the Veteran's Program. Similar to other payors, the government in its role as a healthcare payer needs to assure those that it covers that they are accessing and addressing access to care, quality of care and efficient care. Providers percieve the coverage decisions of the government in a similar fashion to other payors. Providers feel that the payors requirements are disruptive, intrusive, and negatively impacting their patient-provider relationships through burdensome requirements. (McPhillips Deidre. Majority of Americans Don't Trust Government with their Health. U.S. News and World Report. March 26, 2020)

> Samuel is a 71-year-old retired plumber. He had owned his own small family run company for 40 years. We spoke with Samuel about his feelings regarding the government in general, his healthcare coverage through Medicare and then the possibility of a government led single payer system for healthcare. Samuel states that all government officials are out for themselves and therefore he does not trust the government to "work." He shared that when he bought a hammer it cost $20 dollars and not $1200 dollars the government pays." His comment reflected on how poor management and decision making by the government caused him to doubt its ability to manage. He went on to say that he did not trust the government to run a single payer healthcare system. Interestingly, he also talked about how happy he was with his Medicare healthcare coverage not realizing that Medicare is a government run program.

The Affordable Care Act of 2010 (ACA) was the largest healthcare program introduced by the federal government since the Medicare Act of 1965. Initially, many did not trust the government to run this new healthcare program. The reasons for the distrust fell into several categories

1. Those that do not trust the ACA due to partisan ideology
2. Those that feel that the government should not intercede into healthcare
3. Those that feel that the state government is more capable of addressing individuals needs

In the time since the introduction of ACA, its favorability ratings have increased with more people trusting the program. Kaiser Family Foundation statistics have shown that trust and favorability ratings have grown from 40% at its inception to over 55% in 2020. (KFF, 2020) Program attributes such as coverage regardless of pre-existing condition, coverage of individuals up to age 26 in the family policy, coverage of preventative care services and coverage of millions of consumers that were previously uncovered have impacted how consumers see the program. Like many other areas of healthcare, positive experience often leads to an increase in trust. The response of increasing trust and popularity of the ACA is similar to how consumers grew increasingly trustful of the Medicare Part D benefit that began in 2006 through the Medicare Modernization Act of 2003. In addition to positive experience with ACA, an increase in individual self-rated health associated with ACA has positively impacted generalized trust. "Broadening access to healthcare really matters, not only in terms of improved health outcomes, but also regarding positively shaping people's attitudes in general." (Mewes J. Giordano F. Social Science and Medicine, 2017)

Over the last few years, we have seen an increasing number of individuals, both providers and consumers, approving of the government to provide a single national health insurance program. In the last year, more than 63% of consumers have voiced this desire. This is up from 59% in 2019. Only 37% state that healthcare is not the responsibility of the government. This opinion does cut across political lines with an increasing number of independent voters and moderate republicans agreeing with their democratic peers. (Jones Bradley. Increasing share of Americans favor a single government program to provide health care coverage. Pew Research Center, August 2020.)

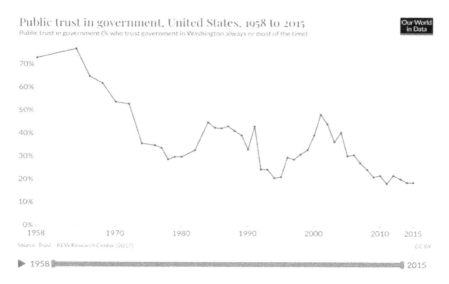

Public trust in government, United States, 1958 to 2015
Public trust in government (% who trust government in Washington always or most of the time)

Source: Trust - PEW Research Center (2017)

## Department oversite

The government's impact on healthcare in the U.S. is not only based on its payor status for approximately half of the consumers in the United States. The government also oversees many organizations that oversee health and healthcare issues including the National Institute on Health (NIH), the Centers for Disease Control (CDC), the Food and Drug Administration (FDA) and CMS to name a few. These organizations often labeled the Federal Public Health System, are responsible for a wide range of activities that support the general health and welfare of the country. These organizations sit under the leadership of the Secretary of Health and Human Services. This position is one of the Cabinet positions that is chosen by the President of the United

States. The activities of these organizations fall into two categories; those that are conducted directly from the federal government which include assessment activities, policymaking, information development and transfer, financing and in some cases direct patient care and those activities that are conducted by state and private organizations.

The actions of these organizations that are either directly or indirectly under the government purview impact multiple stakeholders within the healthcare environment. Due to the importance for the American people, it is important that these activities have no undue influence and are independent of bias. Recently there has been some concern that governmental agencies outside of the public health realm are attempting to place pressure on these organizations to act outside of the best knowledge of science. They are asking the public health departments to ignore their long held "follow the science model". For over 100 years, Americans have trusted organizations such as the CDC and NIH. Unfortunately these recent actions have negatively impacted this trust. Evidence of impropriety will have long lasting impact on the trust of the healthcare agencies within the US government and the decisions that they make. (Baden, September 2020). Research by Brown University Watson Institute for International and Public Affairs showed that consumers lack of trust in governmental institutions has lead to a decrease in the trust of public health intiatives. (Blair, 2017)

## Healthcare Policy

Healthcare policy and regulation are a third area in which both federal and state governments play a crucial role. Many of the policies associated with health and healthcare are promulgated through the agencies that the government oversees. One such example is the Health Information Technology for Economic and Clinical Health ACT (HITECH) of 2009.

The policies and legislation within the HITECH act gave Health and Human Services (HHS) the authority to improve the quality of healthcare through the use of health information technology. The Act also addresses issues tied to health data privacy. Studies have shown the importance of privacy in sustaining trust within the system. Privacy is one of the greatest concerns of consumers. As Hippocrates stated in 377 BC, "things that are holy are reveled only to men who are holy." As more information is tracked and available regarding one's health, there is increasing concern about how this information will be utilized. Consumers regularly articulate their fear of this information being used against them. This is true not only of doctors, insurance companies but also of the government.

More recently, there have been power struggles and arguments made as to who cares about the patient more. It is believed that those creating policy need to better understand the impact of the regulations they put in place. These regulations include reporting, payment and oversite. There have been claims that providers are spending 10-20 hours a week on administrative activities that are mandated through insurance or government.

Many healthcare policies have low visibility to most individuals and organizations. In other cases, healthcare policies can have broad implications across the healthcare stakeholder environment. One such policy is the Trump Administration finalizing the "Transparency in Coverage Rule." This executive Order from the Office of the President is aimed at making health care pricing transparent to the consumer in real time so that they can make informed decisions. This regulation along with the requirements that they set forth for hospitals to disclose their charges including their negotiated rates with third party payers have created a mix of emotions. Healthcare costs are hard to discover and when they are available, they are difficult to decipher. Consumer organizations have applauded these actions while many providers and payers have complained about them.

Ellen is a 49 -year -old woman. Ellen shared her feelings about the transparency of costs in healthcare. "Without my health,

I am nothing. Isn't it interesting that my healthcare is the only place I am unable to get cost information? The government is finally forcing doctors, hospitals and insurance companies to come out and be honest and transparent. All these organizations do is complain and say that it can't be done. Then they wonder why no one trusts them."

James Gelfand, Senior Vice President for health policy at the ERISA Industry Committee stated" the actors charging these prices are doing everything they can to keep prices secret." WoltersKluwer Health found in a survey that they did on price transparency that 87% of hospital executives admitted that healthcare pricing can be cloudy. Transparency policies are great examples of how healthcare policy can have a huge impact on an industry and how it can increase trust in some stakeholders while decreasing trust within others.

A 2019 Pew Study shows that many Americans have a declining level of trust in the country as a whole and more specifically in the federal government and elected officials. They feel that this lack of trust is causing America to be less likely to solve issues focused on healthcare. (Rainie L. Keeter S. Perrin A. Trust and Distrust in America. U.S. Politics and Policy. Pew Research Center. July 22, 2019.) It is important that government officials and the organizations that they lead keep this in mind as they go about their activities. In order to reverse the declining trust that occurs due to these activities, communication, transparency and deeper understanding need to occur. Everyone needs to walk in each other's shoes in order to better understand the other roles, responsibilities and emotions. This is not just true for insurance companies and providers but also government.

"Neither government nor the private sector has succeeded in rationalizing the American health system…when levels of distrust are so high on all sides and in all directions" (Starr P, 2017)

The American Healthcare system sits at the intersection of four important trends; continued decrease in trust both institutionally and personally, significant impact of government of health and healthcare of both individuals and organizations, the increasing discontent in cost, access and quality of healthcare and the unsustainability of the United States healthcare system. The question then needs to be asked, who is the stakeholder most trusted to improve the healthcare system? A 2019 joint study by the Commonwealth Fund and Harvard T.H Chan School of Public Health reached out to healthcare consumers in the United States to ask this question. The answer should not surprise anyone.

The findings include:

1. Providers (Nurses and doctors) were the most trusted individuals but even they are trusted less than would be expected.
2. Nurses were trusted more than physicians as they spent more time with consumers and have better communication skills.
3. The two largest groups that finance a consumers' healthcare in the U.S. are employers and the government. Less than 10% of those surveyed stated that they trust these organizations.
4. Overall, the system did not fare well regarding trust
5. No individual or organization was found to be trusted to improve the system.

# Who do Americans trust "a great deal" to improve the U.S. Healthcare System

| | Percent |
|---|---|
| Nurses | 58 |
| Doctors | 30 |
| Labor Unions | 18 |
| State Government | 14 |
| The Federal Government | 6 |
| Congress | 5 |
| Business Leaders | 5 |
| Health Insurance Companies | 4 |
| Pharmaceutical Companies | 4 |

Source: The Commonwealth Fund/The New York Times/Harvard T.H. Chan School of Public Health, October 2019

This leaves us in a situation where most stakeholders are looking for changes in our healthcare ecosystem but there is no clarity to who should take on the leadership role in making the necessary changes. The lack of trust has placed us in a difficult situation. Who should take the lead? What are the steps that we need to take? How do we start? Trust needs to be earned by all; it takes time.

In speaking with each of the healthcare stakeholders we found that each group believes that they are doing the "right thing for the patient" and warily questions the motives of others. They also believe that they are acting in a trustworthy manner in order to achieve shared goals. We need to move to a world of "positive intent" as this is the only way that trust can be established.

# SECTION THREE:
# TRUST RESETS

"We know it pays to be mindful of trust because it's much easier to destroy than it is to build back up after its' eroded.
Cary Funk, Pew Research Center

# Factors that Impact Trust: Trust Resets

**Trust is like the air we breathe. When it is present nobody really notices. But when it is absent, everybody notices.**
**Warren Buffett**

Trust degradation is not a new phenomenon. It has been occurring for several decades. Overall, the decrease in trust is global but it exists, to a greater degree, in the United States. Experts researching trust have stated that the U.S. is in a trust crisis (Shore). The reasons for this situation are multifaceted. Some of the basic preambles that our country was based on discourage a sense of shared responsibility. The foundation of the United States was built on individual freedom. This belief often collides with the idea of fraternity, equality and solidarity that form the culture of many other countries. In addition, research has shown that specific events that have occurred in the United States have had a lasting impact on trust occurring between governments, organizations, and individuals. Trust is a dynamic process. Trust responds to changes in the environment and one's experiences. It is not written in cement.

An Atlantic Magazine article spoke of moments of "moral convulsions". Each of these moments and events create deep emotions and impact trust affecting a significant portion of Americans. The moral convulsions that create trust resets™ go as far back as the revolutionary period of the 1760s. The trust issues that are created during these times are frequently focused on governmental and institutional organizations, but this is not always the case. Many times these trust resets™ have a more sweeping impact on social trust. Social trust is often defined as whether people or organizations will do what they are expected to do and do what is right. Social trust can permeate all interactions that an individual has. People do not trust that others will have spontaneous sociability. Fukuyama defines this term to mean acting in a way that "sacrifices for the common good". In 1997 64% of Americans had a great deal of trust in United States organizations,

2020 has found this level to have dropped to about 20%. It is not just institutions and the government that Americans distrust, a study done by the University of Chicago found that less than 30% of those surveyed had trust in other individuals. In fact, a large portion of Americans stated that they "don't trust other people when the first meet them." This societal mistrust impacts all facets of life, including healthcare. (Brooks, 2020). Our research shows that there is a lack of trust, not only in our institutions but also between our friends, neighbors and in some cases, even families. The impact of our trust crisis is both deep and wide.

We have chosen four events over the last 60 years to exemplify how trust can be reset. The type of events that initiated the change in trust are different but similar in that they altered trust in a nation for years after the event.

## Events as Trust Resets™

# The Medicare Act of 1965

On July 30, 1965, President Johnson signed a bill focused on health insurance for those over the age of 64. In addition to the Medicare Act of 1965, President Johnson also signed into law the Medicaid program which included both state and federal funding for low- income individuals. President Johnson, when speaking about the Medicare and Medicaid programs, used the Thomas Jefferson statement "without health there is no happiness". This was not the first attempt to create a governmental health insurance program. President Roosevelt considered including one in the Social Security Act of 1934. President Truman tried to pass a national health bill to congress in 1945 and again in the 1950s. He was not successful. President Kennedy had a bill that passed the senate but not the house of representatives in 1964. President Johnson and his two bills were the first time that the government successfully assumed an active role in a national health insurance plan. The Medicare health bill provided hospital and medical insurance for American's senior population. This bill has been extended twice since 1965, once in 1972 to include those with certain disabilities and permanent kidney disease and then again in 2003 to include an outpatient prescription drug benefit.

The American Medical Association (AMA), the pharmaceutical industry, the insurance industry, and others were initially against the Medicare and Medicaid Acts. The criticisms over these programs were loud and, sometimes vicious. All of the industry stakeholders had reasons for opposing these programs. Several stated that the government was creating a socialized medicine program run by communists. In June 1966, a national newspaper ran an article with the headline "AMA Sees Wilber Cohen as Enemy No. One". At the same time, the AMA House of Delagates asked President Johnson to launch a government investigation of Mr. Cohen. Wilber Cohen was the Secretary of the Department of Health and Social Security (precursor to HHS) between 1961 and 1968. He was also one of the architects of the Medicare and Medicaid programs. The AMA had a number of concerns over the programs including governmental interference in the doctor-patient relationship. They called these programs, "government medicine". The insurance industry was not supportive of Medicare because the industry was worried that Medicare would disadvantage existing prepaid medicine programs (later to be called Health Maintenance Organizations) that they sponsored. They were also worried that Medicare and Medicaid would increase the use of hospital services and end up costing the insurance companies large sums of money. (Stevens, Rosemary. Health Care in the Early 1960s. Health Care Finance Review. 1996. 18(2).) The pharmaceutical industry was troubled about the impact of medication use and costs. In response to the anxiety of the industry stakeholders, Wilber Cohen, created the Health Insurance Benefits Advisory Council. This brought together many of those concerned about the new legislation to voice their doubts and find solutions that would make these organizations more comfortable with the governments new role in the healthcare system. In addition, Mr. Cohen publicly and repeatedly stated "that the program would not provide a single medical service... and the government would exercise no supervision or control over the administration or operation of participating institutions or agencies." It was hoped that this would answer the physician's concerns. They also negotiated with the health insurance industry to help reduce their worries by developing commercial insurance carriers to receive consideration as intermediaries for supplemental insurance surrounding the governmental programs. Over time most of the concerns of those within the industry were answered and they began trusting the program. (Berkowitz, Edward. Medicare and Medicaid; The Past as Prologue. Health Care Financial Review 2008 Spring, 29(3)) However, concerns over Medicare and Medicaid remain today. The programs continue to have industry stakeholders that trust them and those that believe that healthcare is not an appropriate role of government.

Although many stakeholders within the healthcare environment did not trust these programs or the government, older consumers and organized labor supported these efforts and trusted them almost immediately. We need to remember that in 1965, over 30% of elderly individuals were living in poverty. In addition, 75% of adults under the age of 65 had some level of hospital insurance, while 50% of those over the age of 65 had no insurance. If a senior needed hospital services, they often looked to others for financial help or went without the needed care. (De Law, N. 2000). The Medicare and Medicaid programs filled a vulnerability for these populations. Rapidly, older Americans and those of lower socio-economic status turned their health and trust over to the government.

Although the government's role in healthcare is still debated, The Medicare and Medicaid programs are trusted by most consumers that rely on them. Studies have shown that the large majority of those covered by Medicare and Medicaid trust these programs. According to a study by Global Strategy Group, 90% of consumers that are covered by Medicare are satisfied with them and trust the programs to cover their health needs. The Medicare and Medicaid Acts of 1965 are a trust reset that has changed the view of government as a healthcare stakeholder forever. Trust in the government and its role in healthcare have continued to evolve. Many trust the government in its role in assisting almost 50% of Americans to receive healthcare benefits while others are leerier. What we do know is that we have recently seen over 60% of consumers voice their desire and trust in the government to make sure that all Americans have health coverage. (Pew Research, October 3. 2018)

## The HMO Act of 1973

Prepaid medical and hospital care has been available for over one hundred years. This form of integrated payment and care was not initially thought of as insurance but as an organizational structure. An example of one such organization is the Pierce County Medical Bureau. Pierce County Medical Bureau was created in 1912 as a cooperative organization between a group of providers and a local fraternal group of lumber workers. The lumbermen had a small amount of their wages deducted to assure medical care when they were injured or ill. Organized medical groups such as the AMA opposed these types of organizations and relationships stating that they exploited physicians. They felt that the pre-paid fixed price model did not align with the services that were given. They felt this type of relationship underpaid and disrespected the participating physicians. This dislike of pre-paid medical care did not recede. The AMA's council on Medical Services stated in 1957 that "All the evils of contract medical practice developed, resulting in lowered standards of medical services, and domination by lay financial interests". This set the stage for the dislike and distrust of physicians as well as others for future pre-paid medical services. (Schwartz, J. 1965)

The 1960s saw a significant increase in healthcare costs. In response to this fiscal challenge, President Richard Nixon passed an amendment to the Public Health Service Act, the HMO Act of 1973. The

Act promoted the development of health maintenance organizations through a number of regulatory provisions. An HMO is a pre-paid insurance plan that integrates financing and care delivery within a given network of providers in a similar manner to the pre-paid medical care that existed in the past. The term "health maintenance organization" was conceived by Dr Paul Ellwood. Ellwood and others believed that if insurance offered a broader set of benefits including preventative care the rising costs of healthcare could be slowed. Proactively addressing healthcare issues prior to them becoming more serious and more costly was a way to achieve this goal. Although there were other aspects to the HMO Act of 1973, the most visible and impactful aspects included the reduced out of pocket costs to the consumer, the covered benefits beyond what was commonly covered in previous insurance and pre-paid plans, and the closed network of providers that would be offering the services and the oversight of services by the HMO.

Prior to the HMO Act, only 2% of consumers had pre-paid medical care. Most of the individuals that had these plans were highly satisfied. The remaining 98% of consumers that were insured had a fee for service model of insurance whereby a limited amount of services were paid by insurance and the remaining services were paid by the consumer. This was a very different payment model than the HMO model and its fixed pre-payment services model.

Although the HMO Act of 1973 began the new era of medical care in the United States, healthcare stakeholders did not really see a significant increase in the HMO model until the mid 1980s. In January 1975 there were 183 HMOs with an enrollment of 6 million consumers. By the end of the 1970s larger national networks of HMOs began to appear. By 1985, the number of HMOs increased by almost 29% to 393 plans and enrollment reaching 25 million members. (Gruber, L. 1988). The early HMOs were offered through non -profit organizations that believed that healthcare could be delivered through quality- controlled medicine which would in turn save money. By the late 1990s, 80 % of managed care organizations were for-profit. It was at this point that the relationships between stakeholders really began to change.

The HMO industry was highly regulated due to the tenets of the law. Healthcare had not previously been as regulated as these new entities. In addition to the increased regulation, the HMO model of care was focused on efficiency and cost. This was new to the healthcare industry and poorly understood. The trust challenge for both the early HMO's in specific and the managed care organizations more broadly, was focused on both the financial and care model that was evolving. This new model created a "lightening rod" of ethical concerns for all the stakeholders. (Gray, 1997) Trust of the model and of the stakeholders involved issues such as:

1. Who had control and was making the decisions regarding the care of the consumer?
2. Did incentive bias create a situation where individuals and organizations were more concerned about their own financial outcome then for doing what was right?

One of the major strategies that was used by HMO plans to address healthcare costs was the use of utilization management. Oversight and control of services was the cornerstone of utilization review. Many believed that the purpose of this activity was to save money. There has been a great deal written about the "fiduciary ethic" and its effect on trust. A fiduciary is a person or organization that is required to act in a responsible manner towards another. Being a fiduciary requires one to act in another's best interest with transparency, integrity and without conflict of interest. Acting as a fiduciary is both a legal and ethical position. This issue was front and center during the period of HMO introduction and the period that followed. Those that were impacted by these actions quickly began to dislike the HMO model believing that all three standards of the fiduciary ethic had been broken. This created a distrust of almost all the healthcare stakeholders who believed that the decision platform utilized by the HMOs was based on the need for the HMO to be profitable and not on the healthcare needs of the consumer.

Prior to the HMO model, the primary relationship in healthcare was between the consumer and their doctor. The entry of the HMO changed this. New models of care, like many new "things" creates concerns and reticence from consumers. HMOs were no different. This was a change that neither party desired. Prior to HMOs, a consumer could choose to go to any doctor that they wanted. Historically, consumers would turn to friends, family, and others that they trusted for physician referrals. Now they were limited in their choice by physician directories associated with their HMO. This limit on physician choice created anger and animosity towards the HMO. Consumers trust in their doctors was tested due to lack of initial choice in the relationship and their frustration in not receiving the care that they often requested. There are studies that found that the early days of HMOs, consumers trusted their physicians less than periods prior to HMO due to this forced lack of choice. The transfer of trust that came from a trusted advisor suggesting a doctor no longer existed. This lack of choice in doctor also created anger and distrust in the HMO as it was their rules that took this choice away. In addition to the lack of choice, consumers were often distrustful of the decisions that their doctors made on their behalf. It was believed by many consumers that HMOs would incentivize their doctors to withhold needed care. This created a concern that self- focused fiduciary goals of the physician were place above consumer need. Consumers were concerned that their providers were more aligned with the HMO and limiting care than supporting the needs of the consumer. There was little focus on the fact that fee for service medicine may have created similar conflicting goals. George Bernard Shaw said this about surgeons "The more appalling the mutilation, the more the mutilator is paid". (Gray,

1997) It was unclear to the patient whether their doctor or the HMO was responsible for the decisions that were being made on their behalf. It was the first time that consumers were hearing the word no regarding care that they felt they needed or wanted. The HMO held little credibility so their saying "NO" caused problems.

Like their patients, healthcare providers were frustrated and mistrusted this new healthcare model. Providers entered contractual relationships with the HMO to participate in their physician network. The contract offered the physician the ability to see consumers that were enrolled in the HMO. Many physicians were unable to continue to see previous patients. This created anger and animosity towards the HMO. In addition to access to patients, these contracts required providers to follow a set of rules. The fear that doctors had previously voiced when Medicare and Medicaid first was introduced once again became a concern. Unlike the Medicare program there were no promises to stay at arms -length and not impact care or the doctor – patient relationship made by the HMOs. To address the increasing healthcare costs in the US, oversight into the care that physicians were giving their patients had to occur. In addition to caring for the medical needs of their patients, physicians were required to take on a new role, that of gatekeeper. Physicians had to get approval from the HMO through the prior approval process to deliver many of the services that they felt were necessary. This form of explicit control of healthcare activities and costs created an additional burden and frustration for providers. To make matters worse, physicians were often prohibited from suggesting services such as tests or treatments that were not covered by the HMO. In addition, they could not criticize the HMO or their rules. Physicians felt that gag rules created a chasm between themselves and their patients. Eventually gag rules were supplanted by state and federal regulations but the damage had already been done. Third- party interference in the patient-physician relationship created distrust in the HMO industry. Doctors did not like HMO due to their loss of autonomy. This third- party interference in the patient-physician relationship created a deep seeded distrust in the HMO industry.

The distrust of the HMO by healthcare providers was not uni-directional. Frequently, the HMO organization distrusted the physicians just as much as the physicians distrusted them. HMO leadership many times felt that the physicians were providing unnecessary care. Some of this was fueled by experience but a great deal more of it was being fueled by the press and other forms of media. (Liu H. Fang H. Rizzo J., HMO and Patient Trust in Physicians: A longitudinal Study. International Journal of Applied Economics, March 2013. 10910 pp 1-21). This distrust often created contentious meetings between the two stakeholders. It was not unusual for HMO executives to bring cost and quality data to a meeting with providers. This data regularly reflected the HMOs concerns over the care that was being given to the consumer member of the HMO. In most cases, there was limited agreement on the data that was being presented and this just furthered the distrust that the HMO had in the provider.

Physicians were not the only providers impacted by the HMOs. Nurses were often replaced by paraprofessionals. Nurses did not trust the rationale that the HMO articulated for making these staffing changes. They felt that this down-skilling of care was financially driven and created significant safety risk to patients. Hospitals were another provider group that were impacted by the HMO movement. A hospital's relationship with both patients and physicians had previously been based on reputation and relationships. The HMO model changed this. Now hospitals had to contract with the HMO entities to be part of the hospital network. This decision limits consumer choice by reducing the availability of hospitals that patients can select from. These contracts often had a significant impact on the revenue model of the hospital as many were required to reduce their fees. In addition, they too were required to receive prior approval for many of the services that they offered including non-emergent emergency department services and hospitalizations. Hospitals felt that HMOs did not treat them as professional healthcare providers, but as a cost center. This lack of respect created distrust and transformed the working relationship between the two entities to one of necessary evil. They were no longer partners.

HMOs and the new models of care did bring with them some good things. They lowered healthcare costs for a period of time and also lowered out of pocket expenses. Preventative care was not only a covered benefit, but it was encouraged. NCQA and other quality organizations were founded, and measurement of healthcare quality was initiated. Evidence based guidelines were implemented and most individuals received an improved quality of care including things such as appropriate medications after a heart attack and a complete set of childhood immunizations.

Regardless of the good things initiated by the HMO movement, the societal outcry against HMOs was loud and very public. Americans were more invested in the consumer and physicians and therefore chose to side them over the HMOS. This created a backlash in the HMOs individually, the HMO model and managed care more broadly. The July 13, 1998 of Time Magazine that asking the question "What Your Health Plan Won't Cover" and the November 8, 1999 cover of Newsweek which said "HMO Hell" say it all. The public did want to see healthcare costs reduced. At the same time, clearly, they did not like the tactics that HMOs used, and the managed care organizations continued. HMO backlash brought with it, increased lack of trust and nationwide proposed legislation, regulation, and lawsuits. In 1996 alone, 56 laws were passed to control the actions of managed care organizations. Many do not remember the good things that came out of the HMO Act of 1973 and the managed care environment. Although the distrust of HMO and managed care has been reduced over the years, a level of distrust in health insurance and managed care remains. The public's lack of trust in HMOs and its re-organization of the healthcare model led to the managed care system's negative reset of trust that still exists in some form today.

## The Terrorist Actions of 9/11 2001

The terrorist attacks in the United States on September 11, 2001 once again created a trust reset™ in the United States. On that day, nineteen extremist militants hijacked four airplanes and attacked the United States. The attack killed almost 3000 individuals. That was not the first terrorist attack that Americans had experienced. The February 26, 1993 World Trade Center bombing, which killed 6 individuals and then the bombing of the Alfred P. Murrah Federal Building in Oklahoma City on April 19, 1995, which killed 163 individuals, both left scars on Americans memory and psyche. The escalating level of terrorism that occurred with the September 11th attack, created an unprecedented level of fear and vulnerability that impacted trust across the United States.

The code of the federal regulations defines terrorism as "the unlawful use of violence against persons… in order to intimidate … and make vulnerable a civilian population". There is no question that one of the many goals of those nineteen individuals that took part in the September 11th terrorist acts was to intimidate and injure the American people. Americans felt vulnerable. As we know, vulnerability and trust are intertwined. When we feel vulnerable, we look to those that can protect us as well as those that can hurt us. September 11, 2001 activated both responses by the American people and created two opposing trust resets.

Politicians and the U.S. government have been found to be the least trusted individuals and institutions as per Edelman. They are perceived as "speaking but not doing" and are unable to provide solutions to the challenges that Americans face. Evaluation of trust in government is often based on whether the "government is doing what is right and perceived as fair". This is considered "political trust". Prior to 9/11 there had been a downward trend in public trust of the government. The summer of 2001, prior to the attacks Edelman Trust Barometer found that only 27% of Americans trusted the U.S. government. The terrorist attacks reversed this trend. By the winter of 2001-2002, trust had risen to 48%. Much of this trust was associated with the "rally around the flag" feelings that often occur when we are pitted against a known or unknown enemy as was the case in the terrorist attacks. The "rally effect" first described by Mueller in 1970 points to the public support and trust when an event occurs that is international, involves the United States and is dramatic. The September 11th attacks were the first significant foreign attack on U.S. soil since Pearl Harbor.

Along with the "us against them" trust impact, was an associated set of emotions including anger and anxiety. Although most terrorist attacks directly impact a small number of individuals, the fear that they create has wide reaching impact. These emotions propagated feelings of vulnerability, loss of control and externally focused anger. The emotional impact of fear and the associated vulnerability leads to an abrupt reaction of trust in the government as the organization that can best protect the population. President George W. Bush created the Department of Homeland Security as a reaction to the terrorist assault. (Ojeda, Christopher. The Effect of 9/11 on the Heritability of Political Trust. Political Psychology. February 1, 2016. 37(1); 73-78). This increased trust due to the attacks impacted consumers views on policies set by the government including policies focused on loss of privacy for individuals and the government reduction in sharing information. Prior to 9/11, most Americans would have been against such policies due to their lack of trust in the government. After the attacks, many Americans changed their views, hoping that these activities would better protect them. This increased trust in government was based on the governments perceived ability to care for and support its citizens. The Brookings Institute called the terrorist attacks of September 11, 2001 a "government moment". The short -lived trust in the government that occurred after September 11th is also not unusual. In most cases, this reactionary type of trust quickly returns to past levels. This upswing in trend directly after the attacks was significant but short lived. One year after the attacks, the trust trend was once again downward. By the winter of 2002-2003 the trust barometer was down almost 10% to 39%. In addition to the increase in trust of the government as an entity, the approval rating for President George Bush rose from 51% to over 90%. The trust and associated approval rating placed in the President was the largest in history. Unfortunately, this increased trust lasted less than a year

The increase in trust during this significant event was not the same for everyone.(Perrin, 2009) (Van Der Does, 2019). While a large portion of the country experienced greater levels of trust in the government, a subset of individuals did not. Easton's statement that trust in government is associated with the government doing what is right and fair came into play for many individuals of middle eastern and/or Muslim descent. This group of individuals felt many of the governmental responses to the terrorist attacks resulted in a feeling of being targeted and not protected by the government. (Government at a Glance, OCED, 2013) The War on Terrorism, felt more like a war on an entire culture, religion and race of people.

Trust in government was not the only change in trust that occurred due to 9/11. Social trust was impacted by the terrorist attacks. Social trust occurs at an individual level. It is important to break down social trust to a more transparent level as the affect was found to be both positive and negative. In cases where trust increased at an interpersonal level the increase was due to individuals relying more on and trusting family, close friends, and neighbors. Understanding the fragility of life increased. More time was spent at home and there was a significant increase in people attending houses of worship. One study found that 19 million Americans rekindled relationships through a variety of communication modalities. (Pew Research Center. Internet and Technology Survey. September 5, 2002). The areas where trust was reduced came from concern and fear over future attacks. (Godefroidt, 2018). Whereas the terrorists involved with the Oklahoma City bombing were Americans, those that were involved in 9/11 were not. These individuals were 'outsiders". Distrust of individuals unlike ourselves is common. As information was provided about the background of the 9/11 terrorists anyone of Middle Eastern or Muslim dissent, or looked similar, was not trusted and was in fact, feared. This ethnic and religious backlash created a significant increase in hate crimes. The FBI and United States Attorney offices investigated over 800 incidents after 9/11 involving violence or threats against individuals perceived to be of Arab or Middle Eastern origin. (United States Department of Justice. 2002). Although the acute level of bias and distrust that occurred directly after 9/11 for individuals of Middle Eastern or Muslim dissent decreased, the trust reset™ of bias towards ethnic and racial minorities remains. (Traugott, 2002)

## The COVID 19 Pandemic of 2020

Trust reset™ events can be local, national, or international. COVID 19 encompasses all three. COVID 19 is the first worldwide pandemic in over 100 years. The outbreak was first identified in December 2019. On January 30, 2020, the World Health Organization declared the outbreak a public health emergency of international concern. This was the same day that the first known case of COVID 19 was identified in the United States. On January 31, 2020, the Trump administration declared a public health emergency in the United States and on March 11, 2020 the World Health Organization declared COVID 19 a global pandemic. By early March the U.S. saw increasing numbers of cases and the US realized that they were in the midst of a healthcare crisis that had serious, even deadly potential for all Americans. The issues associated with trust in others, our healthcare system, the media, and government were all tested. Organizations that many in the United States had never heard of became central for communicating information about a disease that was nonexistent 3 months earlier. Those that we most trusted, our healthcare providers, either lacked information or were unavailable. As this was a new disease, we learned about the disease in real time. All these factors created an environment of "trust reset" ™ that tested the trust in professional competence for all Americans.

The American Psychological Association defines emotion as a "complex reaction pattern, involving experimental, behavioral and psychological elements by which an individual attempts to deal with a personally significant matter or event". Emotions do not have an impact just on an individual, they also have a social impact on how we act and interact with others, including trust.

Consumers level of trust are directly linked to the emotions experienced during COVID 19. Deloitte did a survey of 1159 people approximately 60 days into the COVID 19 pandemic. The survey was focused on the emotional toll that the pandemic had taken on the individuals. The data showed that:

- 82% of individuals had felt anxiety or fear
- 77% of individuals had felt uncertainty
- 75% of individuals had felt loneliness or a sense of isolation

The emotions that Deloitte identified are natural responses when danger or perceived danger exists. In addition to these three emotions, many individuals describe feelings of vulnerability. These feelings are linked to the lack of previous knowledge regarding this new highly infectious disease, the uncertainties surrounding COVID 19, fear of perceived risks for one's self, family, and friends. (Martens, 2020) Emotions can either heighten our need for trust or create barriers to trust. In the case of COVID 19, these emotions created a need for individuals to find those individuals and organizations that they trusted for support and answers. As the pandemic continues to rage on, these emotions have in some cases become barriers to trust.

Esther is a 61-year-old woman who has spent most of her career in retail sales. "At the beginning of COVID, I was scared. I was having nightmares and not sleeping well. I did not know what I could and could not do. Do I go to the grocery store, do I go to my doctor if I get sick? I looked to the news and the experts to give me advice. Here I am six months later, I still am not sure who to listen to and to trust. The fear has not gone away but I have given up trusting anyone. I am just tired and depressed. I am not sure that life will every go back to normal."

Levels of trust have not been stagnant during the pandemic. A Gallup poll found that 36% of those they surveyed stated that they had quite a lot or a great deal of confidence in the U.S. medical system prior to COVID and that it rose to 51% by July 2020. Although the reasons are not clear, it is believed that it is a mixture of the "rally effect" and the media showing the herculean efforts being made by the healthcare system during this time. (Baker, 2020). Consumers emotions, stakeholder's action, increases in communication and political intervention created "trust tides" ™, where trust in different individuals and organizations change based on the fluid nature of the pandemic and its impact. Like other trust reset™ events, the social trust of consumers is being tested during this pandemic. Pew Research looked to identify who individuals trust and rely on for information during COVID 19. They asked consumers the following question: Are people trustworthy, fair, and helpful? (Coronavirus Disease 2019, Trust, Facts and Democracy. Trust in Institutions. Pew Research Center)

- 53% felt that most people could be trusted while 46% felt that most could not be trusted
- 44% felt that most people would try to be fair while 55% felt that most people would try to take advantage of them
- 42% stated that most of the time people would try to help each other while 57% felt that most people were just looking out for themselves

Components of the personal trust scale: Are people trustworthy, fair, helpful?

*% of US adults who choose each response*

**Generally speaking, would you say that most people can be trusted or most people can't be trusted?**

| 53% Most can be trusted | Most cant be trusted 46% |

**Do you think that most people would try to take advantage of you if they got the chance or would try to be fair no matter what?**

| 44% Try to be fair | Try to take advantage 55% |

**Would you say that most of the time people try to help others or just look out for themselves?**

| 42% Try to help others | Just look out for themselves 57% |

Source: Pew Research, March 2020

We asked a set of consumers a similar question; has COVID 19 change your level of trust in others such as your family, friends, or neighbors?

Since the beginning of COVID 19; how has your trust changed in the following groups

Family: 27% decrease
Friends: 15% decrease
Neighbors: 41% decrease
Americans: 57% decrease

Health Intelligence Partners, August 2020

Shelly stated that she found that she trusted her neighbors less. "I see them congregating and not keeping a safe distance from each other as the experts suggest. I understand that Maslow's hierarchy of needs comes into play here. Someone that recently lost their job and is concerned about losing their apartment or being able to pay for food may be less focused on infection control. Intellectually, I understand this. It is just that I am concerned about my family's health and therefore that I do not trust others in my neighborhood to have the same concern. Our vulnerability around health creates a higher standard for me to be willing to trust."

As we dug deeper, we found that this decrease in social trust tended to align with the discordance in beliefs associated with the seriousness and risks associated with COVID. It also in some cases was due to others partisan and political beliefs. Unfortunately, COVID 19 was not the only event occurring during 2020. A contentious presidential election was also in full force during this time and issues around COVID were tightly interwoven with partisan politics. The two events created an overcharged emotional effect on social trust. We found it difficult to dissect the individual components and their impact on trust.

Trust typology associated with COVID 19 has been found to be variable. Initially, much of the focus was on physical trust and the risk of serious health implications to COVID. During its work on trust during the era of COVID, Deloitte has identified four important dimensions of trust which need to be addressed. Each of these dimensions vary depending on the individual's circumstances. As the pandemic has continued, and the impact of the pandemic has broadened, focus has increased on the financial and emotional dimensions of trust. This becomes an important fact as individuals and organizations vie for the trust of both consumer and the organizations that are involved.

**Dimensions of trust: physical, digital, emotional, financial**

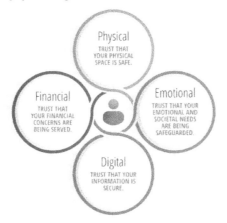

Source: Deloitte analysis.

Deloitte Insights | deloitte.com/insights

In addition to social trust, professional and competence -based trust has been challenging during COVID 19. With any new disease or medical conditions, there are unknowns. We have been learning as we go. This has created challenges in the dissemination of information. As we interviewed people, we heard re-occurring messages such as "The information was conflicting and changing all the time", "all I wanted during that time was for someone to give me advice as to what to do", "afraid I was going to lose my wife" and "My doctor was unavailable". "there was no one that was believable, who was I supposed to trust". "Thank god I have friends that were healthcare workers. They got me basic supplies such as Tylenol, a thermometer, and masks". "Nothing was known but silence and the unknown made it worse". "The information is conflictive and overwhelming and changes every day.' Each of these voices point to a crisis of trust occurring when we feel most vulnerable and afraid.

As we spoke to consumers, there were two overarching themes; the first involves trust in the information while the second focuses on who to trust to get the information. Information has at times been conflicting and at other times has been incorrect and later corrected.

An example of this is the use of face masks to decrease the spread of the disease. Early in the pandemic, it was believed that face masks would not help protect individuals. It was later found that masks did, indeed help. These conflicts and corrections create challenges in the trust of information. ICF, a global consulting services company, has been following public sentiment and trust associated with the pandemic since March 2020. Initially, there was high levels of support for preventative measures to avoid the spread of the virus. (Boyle J. 2020). Unfortunately, due to conflicting messaging, political intervention, and pandemic fatigue some of this support eroded. To counter this challenge, transparency and honesty about the knowns and unknowns is necessary. This has not always occurred. In addition, consumers need to be reminded that during the early phases of a new disease, information may be fluid.

## Personal Measures

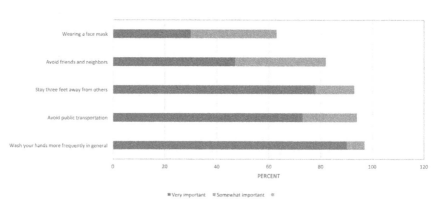

Source: Adapted from ICF Covid-19 Monitor Survey, March 28- April 2, 2020

Trust in health care information during COVID has not only been based on the message but also by the messenger. During the early months of the pandemic, most of the information was being communicated by governmental agencies and the media. Unfortunately, these entities are not highly trusted and therefore important information was often disregarded. In addition, both organizations have been

criticized for being partisan and politically motivated in their messaging. Like other areas where trust has been researched, trust is not
uniform across all populations. Social trust and competence- based
trust during the pandemic has varied by consumer and organizational sociodemographic characteristics, political affiliation, and beliefs
about the pandemic. Men have shown a greater trust in governmental
entities while women have greater trust in health providers and health
experts. (Ali, S. Foreman J, et al. Trends and Predictors of COVID 19
Information Sources and Relationship with Knowledge and Beliefs
Related to the Pandemic: JMIR Public Health and Surveillance. 2020;
6(4); doi: 10.2196/21071)

## Americans have different degrees of trust in COVID-19 information, depending on the source

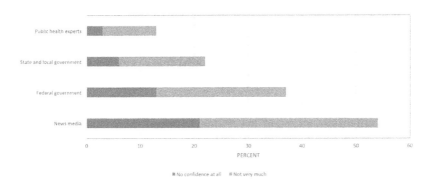

Source: Adapted from ICF Covid-19 Monitor Survey, March 28- April 2, 2020

The second challenge associated with information flow focuses on
who to trust to provide accurate information. Most Americans look to
leaders or those that they have trusted in the past and consult experts
for guidance during a crisis. COVID 19 created several challenges
and opportunities in this area. One such challenge was the lack of
availability of most physicians during the early stages of the pandemic. This left many consumers afloat without their most trusted advisor. Prior to COVID 19, consumers trusted healthcare providers more

than any other group. Unfortunately, consumers found that their providers were often not available during the pandemic due to organizational and financial reasons. Many physician's offices were closed while other physicians that were employed by large provider groups were furloughed. Those providers that were available were learning about the infection while their patients were and therefore had little new information or directions to give their patients. Consumers were unable to get information on topics such as COVID 19 testing and treatment. This created a frustrated and frightened consumer without their trusted anchor. This access challenge and lack of clarity from those that they had previously looked to and trusted created a trust breach™.

> Anton, a 55-year-old male discussed his frustration. "I have cancer and a heart condition. I see four doctors. As COVID 19 began to make the news, I reached out to my doctors. At first, I was able to reach two of them. My heart doctor told me that due to the infection I could not come to his office. He did prescribe extra medicine so that I would not run out. My primary doctor told me that he would be closing his office until this was over and if I needed something I should go to the hospital. I could not reach my other two doctors. Here I was in the middle of treatment for my cancer and being told by the people on TV that I was high risk, and I had no doctor to turn to. I felt abandoned, scared and really mad. Aren't my doctors supposed to be there for me? They went into hiding."

ICF Consulting Strategies and others have reached out to consumers to help identify those individuals or organizations that they trust in receiving this information. In addition to organizations such as ICF, we at Health Intelligence Partners in conjunction with Medecision, a national technology -based care management organization, did our own research. Our research results correlated to that of ICF and others in public health. Health experts were the most trusted individuals during the pandemic, while the national government was the least trusted. In addition, both ICF and our data confirmed that trust in most organizations has eroded since the early phase of the pandemic. This is not unusual and correlates with other significant events where the "rally effect" exists.

## Who are you turning to for information about COVID-19?

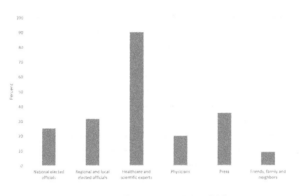

Source: Edelman Trust Barometer, Revive Health Poll

Where do we turn, if not our doctors? As we experience difficult times, either as an individual or a country, we all need to rely on trustworthy individuals and organizations. Several organizations surveyed consumers and found that scientists and health experts have risen to the top of the most trusted category. (Edelman COVID Trust Barometer, Revive Health Poll). Trust in this group of individuals and organizations, including the CDC and NIH, has been relatively consistent throughout the pandemic. Time Magazine named Dr Anthony Fauci, director of the National Institute of Allergy and Infectious Diseases, as one of the most influential individuals of 2020. There were very few weeks we did not hear accolades about this "COVID 19 hero".

Stuart is a middle -aged senior executive. When asked who he trusted for information during the COVID pandemic he shared this," I thought that NIH, the CDC and the World Health Organization (WHO) were antiquated organizations with little real impact on our country and the world until COVID struck. All of the sudden, I realized their importance. They were the only organizations that were sharing science- based information. The scientific and healthcare experts were my go-to people. They took the information from the NIH, CDC and WHO and grounded them in common sense and realism. My doctor who I would have previously trusted was nowhere to be found. The press and the government, both national and local were more entertainment than they were fact based and helpful. I just could not trust their information as they all had ulterior motives."

Our survey found that although scientists have been a trusted source of information since the start of COVID, most recently their trustworthiness has slipped due to conflicting information from different scientists and concerns of political interference. A Kaiser Family Foundation (KFF) poll taken from August 28th to September 3, 2020 found that much of the trust that was created early in the COVID pandemic by the Centers for Disease Control and Prevention and the top scientists and physicians associated with COVID was dropping. The survey found that trust in the CDC has dropped 16 points since the end of April. Forty percent of those questioned feel that the FDA and the CDC are paying too much attention to politics. They feel that these scientific organizations should be free from politics and focus solely on the science. Those that we spoke to stated that they were beginning to wonder if some scientists either were working for the government and therefore were not really following the science or that others may have an investment in the vaccines and therefore were giving advice to bolster their pockets. Early in the pandemic the scientists and public health organizations were looked to for information. We as a country are vulnerable and look to science. Like other times in the past, external factors and lack of trust has impacted issues of trust regarding issues within the healthcare. (Hamel L, Kearney A. The KFF Health Tracking Poll. Kaiser Family Foundation, September 10, 2020) Interestingly, even with this dip, this group is still one of the most trusted sources of information.

Scott Gottlieb MD, MPH and former Commissioner of the Food and Drug Administration (FDA), stated in a Wall Street Journal artilce in April 2021 that it is important for the CDC to keep up with science when making recommendations. He went on to talk about how this alignment of information will help to keep and in some cases, increase trust in public health and public health organizations.

## Percentage of people who say they have a great deal or a fair amount of trust in the CDC

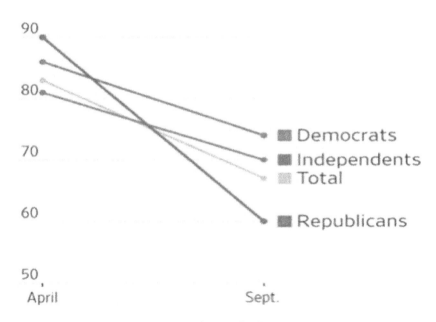

Source: KFF Health Tracking Polls, most recent conducted Aug. 28-Sept. 3 of of 1,199 U.S. adults; margin of error +/- 3 pct. pts.

In addition to scientists and healthcare experts, consumers have looked to their local hospitals to give them advice on the much-anticipated COVID vaccine.

> Suzzana is a 39- year- old mother of two and retail store manager. "They have been there on the front lines of COVID since the beginning. They don't have a financial stake in the vaccine. In fact, if the vaccine works, they will have less patients in the hospital, not more."

Suzzana is not alone in her beliefs. Rob Jekielek, the managing director of The Harris Poll stated, "the organizations that Americans trust most are those who are in the trenches delivering the care". A Harris poll survey taken at the end of August 2020 found that Hospitals and Health Systems were at the top of the list along -side of doctors, nurses, and the CDC.

In addition to healthcare providers, scientists, and experts, we found another group that consumers relied on for information during the early days of the outbreak, employers. Due to quickly evolving changes in the workplace, CEO and HR executives at many peoples' workplace became the "communicator in chief" for information regarding Covid 19. Those surveyed found that employers were more prepared than the government. (62%). In addition to communications, employers worked with their health plan and pharmacy benefit manager vendors to address access and care issues impacted by the pandemic.

COVID 19 has had a significantly positive impact on two groups that previously were found to have low trust levels in the public. Many stakeholders within the healthcare environment believed that these organizations were more focused on their financial successes than on their impact on consumers. Recent trust surveys have found that although health insurance companies and pharmaceutical companies have been the least trusted organizations in health care in the past, COVID 19 has changed this. Consumers have not had a great deal of trust in health plans. Interestingly, their actions during COVID have reversed some of the distrust. By changing rules that were previously in place, 51% of consumers stated that their health plans acted in a way that gave them a level of confidence in being able to get care during this high anxiety period. Consumers stated that health plans had responded with empathy. They went on to say that they hope that this level of empathy will remain after the pandemic subsides. (Deloitte)(Giuliani, S. Will Organizations trust health care organizations after COVID 19 ?, Deloitte Blog May 5, 2020) In addition to health plans, pharmaceutical companies have often found themselves at the bottom of the trust barrel. Prior to Covid 19, only 32% of Americans surveyed had a positive view of the pharma industry. In fact, only government and the tobacco industry had worse trust scores. (Bulik , 2020) A Harris Poll done between April 11 to 13, 2020 found that the pharmaceutical manufacturers reputation since the onset of the virus has increased. Forty percent of those questioned state that they have a more positive view of the industry than before COVID 19. Pharmaceutical companies' ability to help develop and manufacture medications and vaccines places them in both a necessary and important role during the pandemic. John Lamattina, in an April 30, 2020 article in Stat compared pharmaceutical companies' role in manufacturing penicillin during World War 2 to their role today with COVID 19. "They have the potential to save the lives". Axios/Ipsos Coronovirus Index found that trust in the pharmaceutical industry increased from 35% up to 43% in September as news of vaccine success increased. It is now up to the pharmaceutical companies to maintain this new level of trust. Are they able to go back to the days in which they were some of the most admired and trusted organizations? Will their success in creating important new discoveries be overshadowed by the talk of greed?

Whereas the health plan and pharmaceutical industry have increased trust during this pandemic, journalism and journalists have found themselves challenged in many ways. Early in the pandemic, Americans relied heavily on the news media for information. Nielson rating skyrocketed during the month of March. Fox News had its most watched week in its history from March 16-22. They were not alone. CNN was up 1515% during the same time period. Mainstream and social media became the most relied on source of information with those over 55 years old relying on news media more whereas younger consumers relied on social media (56% verse 54%). Unfortunately, this significant utilization of the media as a means of receiving information has not translated into trust of the information. We need to ask why they are the most relied upon but not the most credible or trustworthy. Media, regardless of the source is the most easily accessed information, but as we stated earlier in the book, many consumers feel that news has become "infomercials and entertainment" more than factual. Mertens and his co-authors found that there was a link between media exposure and fear. (Martens, 2020) Many people feel that the fear is not due to the facts, but because of the sensationalism that today's media is based on. Sensationalism sells.

In addition to the sensationalism, studies have found that there is an overarching concern about "fake new and biases associated with political viewpoints. Axios found that 62% of Americans don't trust media and news due to "fake news".

> Jorge, a 44-year-old individual stated that, "I grew up trusting the people that did the news, today they are at the mercy of ratings and advertising. They are here to sell us something, not to tell us something." Jorge went on to share that "all newsmen are pawns. I don't care the channel. They are political messengers that lie."

Considering the current lack of trust in news and media which supplies a significant amount of information about COVID 19, it is unsurprising that consumers distrust much of the information that they are receiving about the pandemic.

Media is not alone when it comes to the trust challenges that we are living through. Government has consistently been the least trusted source of information during this pandemic. 85% of consumers stated that they wanted to hear more from the scientists such as Dr Anthony Fauci and less from the government. Only 20% of consumers said that they trusted the government to help fight the virus. (Edelman). ICF, a global consulting services company found that local governments have been a more trusted source than national government. There are some states and cities where local governments are considered trustworthy. Unfortunately, consumers sentiment seems to be finding decreasing trust in both local and national government. The reasons for this vary but seem to point to the vitriolic and polarizing talk from those in charge. Several people shared their belief that the representatives of the government are more concerned about their re-elections than serving their constituents. One other reason for the lack of trust at the national level is the conflicting information provided by our national leaders, information contradicted by many scientists (remember, scientists have been the most trusted group during COVID 19.) The rally effect that occurred directly after the 9/11 attacks did occur to a degree very early in the pandemic. This was seen for both national and local governmental agencies. Large number of Americans watched President Trumps COVID task force daily. Governor Cuomo was not only watched by citizens of New York but nationally. His favorability rating increased for both democrats and republicans. Governor Cuomo utilized both transparency and empathy during his daily updates. He recognized that these attributes are necessary to reduce the emotional impact of COVID and gain trust during these times. He focused not only on health but also about well- being including things such as job, financial, housing and food security. His empathy created a "shared or collective identity" which improves trust. It becomes an "us versus them", with the "them" being the virus and not each other. It was a great example of the "rally effect" model. Unfortunately, the rally effect quickly diminished. A survey done between August 7 and August 26, 2020 found that early in the pandemic there were increased levels of trust in the government to be able to effectively lead the American people through the pandemic. This "rally effect" of trust has decreased significantly from late April to August. (Baum M. Lin J. et al. The State of the Nation: Public Trust in Institutions and Vaccine Acceptance. September 2020. Doi. http://www.kateto.net/covid19/COVID19%20CONSORTIUM%20 REPORT%2013%20TRUST%20SEP%202020.pdf)

## Do you trust the information you hear about the coronavirus (COVID-19) from...

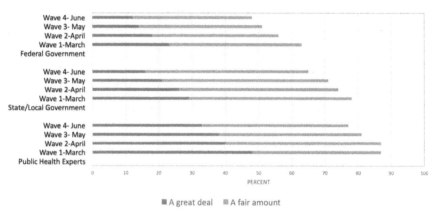

A great deal · A fair amount

Source: ( Adapted from ICF analysis using Mfour data collected from a nationwide sample from March 28-June 29, 2020)

The impact of this regression of trust is potentially significant as we begin the process of immunizing Americans against the virus. In July, 66% of those asked said that they would receive the vaccine when it becomes available. By September, that number has decreased to 59%. Although it is not unusual for the rally effect to lessen over time, in the case of the COVID 19, the impact was very short lived. Some of this reduction in support and trust was based on partisan and political viewpoints. In other cases, it has been due to the conflict between the information that is being distributed by the government politicians and what individuals are experiencing. Governmental entities that stated publicly that "everything was OK" and that the virus was not dangerous. At the same time, individuals were getting sick at alarming numbers.

The trust reset™ associated with the COVID 19 pandemic are numerous. First, is the fact that the United States healthcare system is based on sick care and not on prevention. Public health in this country is at best an afterthought. There is hope that one trust reset™ will include renewed focus on public health and prevention. A second trust reset™ is focused on the importance of information. The proliferation of healthcare misinformation has significantly affected consumer trust in messaging and the messenger. World Health Organization has called the information regarding the pandemic an "infodemic"

The importance of communicating accurate, transparent, and honest information is the lesson that needs to be learned from this period. (Lee, 2020) John Barry, the author of The Great Influenza said " In the next ....pandemic, be it now or in the future, the single most important weapon against the disease will be a vaccine. The second most important will be communication." (Lee, Nov. 2020.) In conjunction with information is the trust reset™ associated with the overlap of politics and healthcare. The U.S. is not the only country where healthcare solutions are impacted by political beliefs, but it is a country where the rhetoric and power positioning made a significant impact on the health of its citizens. COVID 19 has demonstrated the importance of science being trusted by individuals, organizations, and the government. For government to create good policy it needs to utilize good science.

There are two other healthcare related trust resets™ that will occur as a factor of the COVID 19 pandemic. The first is the use of virtual care. The use of virtual care more than doubled during the pandemic. In addition, 80% of those that utilized this method of healthcare stated that they were satisfied with the care and would trust this method of care in the future. They also stated that whether it was virtual visits with family, friends or a member of their healthcare team, this mode of interaction reduced the feeling of abandonment or isolation.

The trust tides that we have spoken will create changes in levels of trust as we continue to battle the pandemic and, in the post-pandemic era. Organizations will have to be prepared to address the perceptions and realities of the COVID impact and ask themselves what they did right and what they did wrong. Those organizations that gained in trust with others will have to decide what they can do to maintain that trust. Will health plans remain more consumer focused and flexible? Will pharmaceutical companies reset the conversation towards science and away from costs? This once in a century pandemic trust reset™ event has lessons in trust for all of us regardless of one's role during COVID 19.

## Fifteen Actions that Create "Trust Resets" ™

The United States is at a crossroad. Conversations about overhauling the healthcare system grow louder each day. The reason, lack of trust. There is little disagreement that there needs to be changes in healthcare and that transformation needs to occur. There may be disagreement on whether the changes include financial, organizational, policy or governmental changes. The truth is that without trust, none of these changes will successfully move the American system to where it needs to be. The reality is that trust does not exist within the healthcare system today. Robin Hochstatter, a healthcare consumer stated "Trust has rusted from the inside out. We did not realize that the rust was occurring until it crumbled and took the healthcare system with it." Warren Buffet, an American business magnate stated that "Trust is like the air we breathe When it's present, nobody really notices but when it is absent everybody notices." The lack of trust has placed us in an untenable situation. We continue to ask; Who should take the lead? What are the steps that we need to take? How do we start? Trust needs to be earned by all; it takes time. As Arthur Ashe stated:

> Start where you are.
> Use what you have
> Do what you can

> Arthur Ashe 2016

The first step is to understand that trust must be earned. Some people feel that trust is automatic, largely based on power or given because we have no other option. This is not the case. Trust is fragile and hard to regain after being lost. Like the nursery rhyme about humpty dumpty, trust is hard to put together again. We surround ourselves with people that reflect our beliefs, a community either real or virtual. Discordance can create distrust of both parties, but it does not have to. The power of trust needs to come from numerous places. There are many things that can impact trust and change trust. Trust in our current world is being jostled around like a set of dice in a Yahtzee game. Yes, in many ways trust has been lost in healthcare today. The good news is that trust can be regained.

As was stated in the Revive Trust Survey, trust has a number of attributes. Like a garden, there are many factors that contribute to its growth. Trust can be tested, potentially bruised but if we agree on its importance and focus on our role it will again become the strong foundation of healthcare. We are going to look at a number of reasons that trust has been tested, potentially bruised, and occasionally lost. These trust reset™ actions include institutional factors, individual factors and behaviors and psychological factors. Dr. John McEnery was a pediatrician in Oak Park Illinois in the 1970s taught every pediatric resident that he worked with that the most important tools that a pediatrician had in caring for their patients were trust, compassion, and knowledge. Our research has found that there are 15 trust resets™ that form the basis of re-engaging and rebuilding trust.

Steps to accomplish the trust reset™

## 1. Accountability and responsibility

How often have we heard the comment "it's not my decision or not my job"? How do these statements make us feel? Angry? Frustrated? Unclear accountability and responsibility can create unhealthy and untrustworthy relationships both within an organization and across stakeholders. In order to build a trusting relationship, it is important for each individual or organization to understand their role. Internally, redundancy of roles creates unhealthy competition within an organization. Instead of ensuring that goals are met, it often leads to unhealthy competition, destructive relationships, and lack of trust. All parties need to understand what they are responsible for.

External clarity of responsibility is equally problematic. It is not unusual to hear someone in healthcare ask "who is in charge" or "who is the decision maker?" This "passing the buck" leads to the perception that someone is trying to hide something or purposefully making something difficult. Lack of clarity breeds confusion, frustration, and distrust.

Recommendations:

- a. Individual:
    - i. Each of us has a role to play, understand your role and responsibility, whether you are a consumer, healthcare provider or other professional.
    - ii. If you are unsure, get clarification regarding roles and responsibilities. This will help in the interactions that you have with others and increase bi-directional trust. It will also increase the likelihood of a positive outcome.

b. Organizational:
   i. Corporate understanding of each individuals and divisions roles will improve working relationships.
   ii. Titles, roles, and responsibilities vary across organizations. These differences can create unreasonable expectations which can lead to distrust. Document roles when possible.
   iii. Agree on what each organization brings to the table.
   iv. Do not create redundancy in responsibility. This is especially important in organizations that have a matrixed reporting system.
   v. Document roles and responsibilities and review this on a regular basis. This can be done through the use of checklists or other tools.
   vi. When possible create a "one touch resolution" within the organization.

## 2. Bias

Each of us has a history and a background that forms a basis of who we are and what we believe. This history creates beliefs and experiences that impact how we interact with each other. This is true not only in our general daily actions but in all of our health care interactions as well. Past actions have created deep distrust of the healthcare industry. Experiences by many individuals has been tainted with the paint brush of medical racism. Although the Tuskegee Study of untreated syphilis occurred from 1932-1972, ongoing racism and personal experiences has continued to propogate mistrust within the Black community. Evelynn Hammonds, a Harvard historian said, "disparity is built into the healthcare system" Ongoing distrust of Muslims and others of Middle eastern descent since 9/11 continues. Bias and prejudice are part of our history and still exists in today's environment. We are living in a polarized country today that is creating heightened levels of stereotypes and bias. These need to be recognized but they are not written in stone. Most people tend to trust those that are most like them because that is who we are most used to interacting with. This behavior itself, is based on bias.

Biases, stereotypes, and prejudice impact how individuals interact. This is true whether they are based on demographic characteristics, job title or organization. All individuals have bias. In some cases, it is acknowledged and in other cases it is not. These views, whether perceived or real, propagate further bias and create distrust.

Regardless of whether they are conscious or unconscious, biases can be destructive in a number of ways, including damaging relationships, poor experiences, poor outcomes either business or clinical and inequality within healthcare. Recognition of past actions and issues increases distrust. We need to admit that there are biases and address them. This act alone, can improve trust.

Bias is found in many different circumstances. It can be found in a clinical interaction originating from either the provider or the patient. A 2017 national survey, The Patient Prejudice Survey; When Credentials aren't Enough, found that 60% of the 1,000 healthcare providers surveyed had experienced bias. These experiences included offensive remarks about age, race, gender, or ethnicity. (Tedeschi, 2017). Over 90% of the providers stated that these negative interactions impacted their trust in their patients.

It can also occur in the healthcare executive suites. Minorities fill only a small minority of C-suite and board positions. In many of these cases, they are considered the "token" and lack respect from others in similar positions. In our conversations with minority executives, we found common themes; "we have to work twice as hard to be respected half as much", "when someone is hostile I have to keep my mouth shut if I want to keep the job", "when someone tells a bigoted joke, I feel like I have to laugh along in order to feel like a member of the board."

Recommendations:

    a. Individual:
- i. Be honest with one's self and with others. We all have unconscious bias. Recognize it and focus on seeing people as individuals. Interact with them with respect and consideration.
- ii. Broaden your belief and demographic interactions.

    b. Organizational:
- i. Corporate leadership needs to take a public role in addressing bias. This will impact both individuals within and outside of an organization.
- ii. In order to eliminate bias, leadership must take deliberate steps.
- iii. The first and probably one of the most important is to hire a diverse workforce.
- iv. Forums for open dialogue are important. Create opportunities for employees to interact with individuals of different demographics and thought processes in a safe space. We won't always agree but differing views need to be discussed. These activities are well worth the time and effort.
- v. Implement structural changes and create systems and on-going training.
- vi. Create broad diversity policies and regularly benchmark yourself and organization against those policies. Look externally to identify best in class practices in diversity and anti-bias practice
- vii. Consider hiring a Chief Diversity Officer. This role does not remove the responsibility of increasing diversity and decreasing bias from the CEO. The role is to assure continuous vigilance and improvement.
- viii. Create working relationships with other organizations that are addressing bias and discrimination.

ix. Identify partners that are trusted within different cultures, races, and religions such as places of worship, community centers, salons, and stores.

### 3. Communication

Communication is foundational in all relationships and can be a positive or negative trust reset™. Trust cannot occur without some type of relationship. Communication is the key to a strong and lasting relationship. Communications has been shown to be one of the most important aspects of any relationship whether it be between a provider and their patient, between healthcare workers (Kelly Michaelson) or the interchange between healthcare executives. Of those that we surveyed, over 75% stated that they trusted their provider because of "how they talk to me". Communication between individuals is like a dance. Sometimes it is clunky and other times it is graceful. As Kelly Michelson found "open lines of communication, open the gates of trust". Good communication is not one sided. In addition, effective communication includes both verbal and non-verbal components. Communication is based on a number of factors; information sharing, respectful and humble questioning and listening.

There are several attributes that should be considered when one is focused on creating a positive trust reset™ in communication. One important aspect of communication is consistency. Inconsistency in messaging creates distrust. When there is inconsistent messaging those receiving the information do not know who to trust and, in many cases, end up not trusting anyone. This has been shown to be the case early in the COVID pandemic in regard to mask wearing and methods of spreading of the virus.

Means of communication can also be a trust reset™. Face to face, phone, email, text, or other forms of social media can be utilized. Although all modalities can be effective, face to face communications have the greatest positive impact on trust. Face to face communication allows for the use of body language including shows of compassion, active listening, and facial expression. The act of "showing up" communicates respect. If an in-person meeting is unfeasible, a digital face to face can accomplish some of the same things. The primary alternative to face to face through the COVID 19 crisis is video. If neither of these alternatives are available, the next most effective trust building means of communication is voice communications. People are more likely to engage in small talk. Small talk or "social cement™ leads to stronger relationships and trust.

A second important aspect associated with verbal communications focuses on the use of jargon. It is not unusual for someone to unconsciously use jargon. The use of words that others do not understand creates a wedge in the relationship. It can also be perceived as a form of disrespect. The Moments in Truth research report of 2016 found that for 69% of healthcare consumers healthcare jargon was a significant barrier to trust and their ability to actively participate in decision making regarding their care.

Edgar Schein, in his book, Humble Inquiry, divides verbal communication into telling versus asking. In the United States, we are often taught that telling is the most important and respected form of communication whereas in other countries, questioning is often more respected. Inquiry, in all its forms is a cornerstone of a communications- based relationship. Asking questions shows others that you are interested in them and their thoughts. It also reduces the likelihood of incorrect assumptions. When interacting with others in the healthcare environment, it supports clarifying desired needs and goals. A survey of 2000 adult consumers found that they want to discuss more than just their physical health with their doctors during a visit. Patients wanted to discuss their goals for health and things such as happiness and for older adult's issue such as independence and well-being. These patients talked about how physicians mainly focused on symptoms and physical health. These consumers are looking for their relationship with their doctor as holistic. (Sarah Heath) Talking past each other is in direct conflict with relationship building. By asking someone a question, you are "inviting them into the conversation." Baker, 2020) In addition, humble inquiry is a sign of respect. You are looking for their thoughts and opinions. A third aspect of inquiry or question asking that destroy trust is when we ask a question and we really do not want an answer. I call this the "doorknob" question. Asking a question, while standing at the door with your hand on the doorknob conveys through body language you lack desire for a response. It also shows a lack of respect for the potential response of the other individual. This action is a clear negative trust reset™.

"Doorknob" body language is a good example of the importance of non-verbal communication. We often do not realize that our body language speaks as loudly as our words. Mehrabian in his research found that the "silent messaging" of non- verbal communication can impact trust. Things such as facial expression, eye contact, body positioning such as sitting forward in an engaged fashion and not looking at your watch or phone can positively impact a relationship. Subtly mirroring another's gestures can also convey empathy which leads to increased likelihood of trust.

Communication is not just speaking but also listening. Consumers feel that their providers don't have the time to listen to them, that they are "stuck on a profit driven treadmill" (Walker, 2019). Dr. Robert Gatson taught me that listening is more important than speaking. Individuals want to be heard. Ask questions. Khullar and his fellow authors talks about "listening with humility". An example of the challenge to listening is the story of Joe. Joe was battling a serious cancer. He was given a new medication prescription from his doctor and told to have the prescription filled at a retail pharmacy. The medicine had serious side effects including risks to unborn infants. When Joe went to the pharmacy, the pharmacist, who never looked up asked Joe if he was pregnant. Joe laughed and said no. As Joe's wife shared with me, Joe no longer went to that pharmacy because he did not trust them. First, they did not engage Joe in an appropriate manner and secondly, they did not listen, really listen. Listening is an important factor in communication. "even through silences." It shows that you care and humanizes both you and the other party. Listen to what the other party is saying. Acknowledge whatever emotion that a patient and their family may have. This is important for any provider (doctor, nurse, pharmacist, and hospital staff). Numerous studies have found that providers wait only about 11 seconds before interrupting a patient after asking a question. Listening is also important in the executive suite. It is not unusual an executive to be thinking about what they want to say instead of actively listening to the answer of a colleague. Even worse, is the common action of looking at one's emails or text messages while someone else is speaking. Good active listening skills are a way to show that we are taking what others say seriously. It is a form of respect that leads to strong relationship building.

Education is an area in which communication can help to build a trusting relationship. Admitting ignorance places an individual in a vulnerable situation. How another party reacts to that admission can be an either a positive or negative trust reset™. Non-verbal communication through open body, eye contact, not acting rushed, and active listening gives the questioning individual the opportunity to actively participate in the educational process. Verbal communication skills including speaking at a reasonable pace and using words and concepts that the other individual will understand, allowing for successful transfer of information. David Schleifer surveyed a group of individuals with chronic medical conditions. Those surveyed articulated the importance of the doctor taking the time to educate them and answer their questions. Our research found similar findings. One consumer stated that "I know that my doctor is busy, but he took the time to make sure that my wife and I understood what we needed to do in order to keep me healthy. My wife always has lots of questions and he did not rush us. He told us that no question was stupid. I will trust him to do the right thing in the future because he showed he cared and wanted us to really understand."

    a.  Individual-
- a. It is important that everyone practice good communication skills. This includes understanding the importance of both verbal and non-verbal skills. Don't assume that your communication skills are as effective as we would like.
- b. Whenever possible, utilize face to face communications early in a relationship. This leads to stronger relationship building and greater trust
- c. Healthcare is full of jargon. It is important to avoid using jargon. We often do not even realize that we are using words that others may not understand. Understanding and practicing health literacy is important for understanding as well as showing respect to others. This has been used by international organizations to help understand verbal and non-verbal skills associated with cultures around the world.
- d. Be aware that different cultures have different communication styles. Utilize resources such as Kiss, Bow or Shake Hands by Terri Morrison as a tool.
- e. Learn how to ask questions in a respectful way. Humble questioning and inquiry are a valuable skill and one that consciously needs to be practiced.
- f. Remember to use active listening skills.
- g. Put away your cell phones and computers during conversations with others.
- h. Make sure that you make enough time for conversations. If time is short, acknowledge it and set a time for further conversation
- i. Private communications should occur out of earshot from others. Hallways, restaurants, elevators, and other public

spaces are not appropriate locations to have most conversations. You never know who is listening or who may be standing next to you.

    j.   Communications which include "small talk", or "social cement" help to create relationships and increase trust. Make time for this type of communication

b.  Organizational:

    a.   Develop and/or offer educational tools and resources to support effective creating communication skills for your employees. Be conscious of jargon differences between stakeholders

    b.   Educate employees of cultural communication differences

    c.   Utilize conscious scheduling of meetings. This can include meeting times aligned with interaction need and providing 10- minute breaks between meetings.

    d.   Create policies regarding computer and cellphone use during meetings

    e.   Display reminders regarding conversational privacy in key public areas

    f.   Utilize face to face meetings whenever possible. If individuals are in the same building, have all individuals attend in person.

## 4. Compassion and Empathy

"Stop looking at scores. Start loving"
Julie Kennedy Oehlert, the Chief Experience Officer at Vidant Health

Empathy is the ability to sense another's feelings and therefore respond in a manner that is both appropriate and engaging. Empathy requires us to be willing to be open and engage with others. Showing empathy can both build and maintain a relationship. The phrase "before you judge a man, walk a mile in his shoes" is a reminder of what we need to do in order to practice compassion and empathy. It not only allows for one to be aware of another's feelings but also to have a better understanding of the other person's needs. Think about the Ritz Hotel experience where the front desk staff comes out from behind the desk. This form of engagement allows for increased trust between individuals and teams.

Communication is an important tool in showing both empathy and compassion. This can be done through an individual's tone and voice quality, volume, and speed of speech. (Mehrabian, 1981). In addition, compassion and empathy are achieved through listening. Without these skills, empathy and compassion are not always felt to be genuine.

Compassion and empathy are important aspects in creating a trusting provider and consumer relationship. A Managed Care Executive study found that consumers no longer want a relationship tied to a "title" or credentials, they want one 'rooted in empathy". They are looking for an on-going relationship with a trusted provider, one who cares". (Walker 2019) Trust is impacted by the patients' perception that their physician or others within the healthcare system care and are empathetic to their needs. One study found that 57% of consumers believe that their doctor cares about them most of the time, 33% some of the time, 9% none of the time.

Although most providers believe that they are compassionate and empathetic individuals, some find it difficult to express empathy. This does not mean the provider is not empathetic, but it sometimes is felt by the consumer that the doctors are not empathetic and do not care about them. Survey found that 71% of those asked stated that their doctors did not show compassion or empathy during the visits. This feeling has a negative trust reset™ impact on the trust between the provider and consumer.

Anthony Orsini, a neonatologist understood the importance of empathy and compassion in regard to trust. He also understood that many doctors do not show compassion. He created tools for doctors to use in order to better communicate compassion. The Orsini Way focuses on the fact that "when you truly care, you truly connect". He sees this as a method to help physicians to help build trust "The Orsini Way" addresses the challenges that doctors have in regard to compassion including:

1. Lack of training to communicate effectively and compassion-ately. It focuses on both verbal and non-verbal skills such as reminding doctors to look into the patient's eye and not at the computer screen, using open ended questions, not interrupt patients, and utilizing active listening skills.
2. Reminds doctors that although they are task oriented, inter-acting with their patients in a compassionate and empathetic manner will help them to achieve those tasks. Only a few ac-tions and words are needed to make a big difference.

Compassion and empathy are also important in the non-clinical set-ting. empathy has been shown to increase respect. One in three work-ers have said that they would leave their companies for somewhere that is more compassionate as they don't feel supported and do not trust the company. This is especially true in younger adults. In addition to building individual relationships and trust, empathy and compassion have been found to between build strength and a sense of community in cross functional teams. (Businessolver 2017 Workplace Monitor).

Recommendations

a. Individual
   a. Listening skills are a key to empathy and compassion. Make sure that you are not distracted while listening to another.
   b. Start each conversation by asking people how they are and give them the time to answer. These few minutes will be well worth it

        c.  Utilize open ended questions during conversations, you will learn more about the individual.

    b.  Organizations
        a.  Empathy requires an organization wide effort.
        b.  Leaders of organizations need to understand that people are the key to success. Creating an empathetic and compassionate organization does not show weakness. It actually builds strong loyal teams.
        c.  Modeling empathetic behavior can show the power of empathy towards trust.
        d.  Offer resources to employees on how to practice empathetic behavior.
        e.  For organizations with healthcare providers, companies such as Empathetics help to train physicians in their ability to express empathy.

## 5. Competence

The 2020 Edelman Trust Barometer stated that one of the most important factors that build trust is competence. This is especially true in healthcare both at an individual and at an organizational level. Competence is not just based on education; it is in having the attributes needed to perform a job successfully. There are four components to competence to consider regardless of one's role. They include the knowledge of how to do a job, the skill to succeed, the judgement on how to address a situation and the behavior to effectively manage the situation. Healthcare knowledge can be both technical and operational. Whereas technical is "what", operational focuses on the "how". Operational competence focuses much more on the contextual portion of competence. (Hill L. Lineback K. To Build Trust, Competence is Key. Harvard Business Review. March 22, 2012.)

Competence is shown through both communication and through actions. Competence is not a one- time event, it is a consistent evaluation of one's abilities over time. When someone does not trust the competence of those that they are working with, they tend to either micromanage, not delegate, or look elsewhere for support.

Competence is an important factor in the provider-consumer relationship. Health is one of the most sacred and personal things that each consumer has. When an individual is seeking healthcare from a provider, it is often at a time of vulnerability. The competence of the healthcare provider is an important factor in trusting that provider. It reduces the uncertainty that often is part of a patient's healthcare experience. It also includes the operational competence to have the confidence needed throughout the experience. Earlier in the book we heard from Sasha that equated her doctor's educational pedigree to competence. This still exists with some consumers but there are an increasing number of consumers that look to other attributes to access competency.

The competence that a provider shows focuses on both the ability to diagnose and the skills to treat a patient. Providers, especially physicians, spend many years learning their craft. The Hippocratic oath states that physicians dedicate themselves to "heal the sick and care for the well". Most doctors pride themselves on being competent. This pride sometimes gets in the way of healthcare providers not admitting to themselves or others their lack of knowledge about something. "I don't know" is a hard thing for providers to say. Interestingly, it has been shown that patients do not loose trust in their providers when they admit this. In fact, it can increase trust. It shows that they are confident and have the courage to admit that they don't know. It also depends on how this lack of knowledge is articulated. "I don't know but I will find out and get back to you" can be very comforting to most individuals. It shows vulnerability which increases trust and increases credibility in other issues.

While credibility is an important trust reset™ issue between the healthcare provider and their patient, there are an increasing number of stakeholders in healthcare that are scrutinizing the competency of healthcare providers. It has become increasingly important that healthcare providers demonstrate their competency. Much of the focus is due to the actions of a few. Unfortunately, it has created a negative trust reset™ in certain circumstances. It is important that the criteria for defining competence for healthcare providers be clarified and measurable.

Competency is equally important outside of the provider-consumer relationship. In many cases, individuals and organizations have limited exposure to each other. This creates a situation where competency has to be proven on a regular basis. In addition, the expertise of many of the organizations is known only through assumption, reputation, or perception. This creates a difficult atmosphere for trust to thrive. It is not unusual for a healthcare executive to distrust levels of competency of government officials or providers that are now focused on the business of medicine due to pre-conceived notions. (Nasher) Most organizations come with a technical and/or operational competence to the table that can be valuable to the activity that you are focused on. Use that to create trust in the team.

Recommendations

    a.  Individual
        i.  Healthcare providers
            1.  Maintain your education both formal and informal
            2.  When appropriate, continue with ongoing certification
            3.  Don't be offended if a patient or their family requests a second opinion. In most cases, this does not reflect on your competence.
            4.  Don't be afraid to say "I don't know"
            5.  Don't be afraid to ask if you do not know something, it increases trust of others

    ii.  Non-clinical providers (The recommendations are not significantly different than healthcare providers)

        1.  Maintain your education both formal and informal

        2.  When appropriate, continue with ongoing certification

        3.  Don't be offended if a patient or their family requests a second opinion. In most cases, this does not reflect on your competence.

        4.  Don't be afraid to say "I don't know"

        5.  Learn how to power talk (Nasher, 2018). Women need to recognize "powerless speech" and overcome it.

  b.  Organizational

    i.  Don't let bias or assumption impact beliefs in others level of competency

    ii.  Create definitions of competency that are clear and measurable if possible.

    iii.  Skills don't always speak for themselves, give others the chance to demonstrate competence either through action or behavior.

    iv.  Require and monitor licensing and ongoing certification where appropriate

    v.  Create a culture where qualified individuals are practicing at the top of their credentials

    vi.  Support on going educational opportunities in order to create a culture of life -long learning and competency.

## 6. Consistency

Trust is not a "one and done". It occurs over time. Think about a restaurant that you enjoy going to; why do you enjoy it? We asked that question to a number of individuals. Some stated that they liked the ambiance, others said the service and a third group said the food. One thing that they all said was that they knew that each time they frequented the restaurant they trust the experience would be good. This consistent experience led to trust. Unfortunately, we live in an inconsistent world. This is one reason that we struggle trust across our daily lives.

Consistency in interactions regardless of the industry is important. Consistency in action, in words and in temperament all play an important role in healthcare. Lack of consistency is often equated with not caring or lack of respect. There is a reputational impact as well as a trust impact. Regardless of whether it is a clinical interaction between a provider and consumer, or a business -based interaction, inconsistency decreases the likelihood that we will be trusted by others or that we will trust others.

Consistency is not just doing the same thing or acting the same way during each interaction, it is also aligning and being consistent between words and actions. Do what you say you will do. We heard from the surveys that consumers lost trust in their providers after the provider made a promise to call and then did not follow up. This was not only articulated regarding the clinical interaction, but also articulated in regard to health plan follow up.

In the end, consistency removes the uncertainty that can create a negative trust reset™ and creates a positive reputation.

Recommendations

1. Individual
    1. Consistency can be tied to creating good habits It has been shown that habits lead to routine which in turn leads to consistency
    2. Keep your promises, consistency between words and actions are important
2. Organizational

1. Be aware of activities and organizational makeup that create inconsistencies in your organization.
2. Create expectations of consistency through policies and procedures
3. Identify measurable data points that identify inconsistencies within your organization. Review and rectify on a regular basis.
4. Align employees and corporate brand and goals. People work with people and not organizations. Your employees need to represent the organization

### 7. Costs and other financial issues-

Finances and costs are well- known causes for negative discourse within a family. (Holland, 2015) In fact, it is second most common cause for divorce according to Ramsey Solutions. Costs and financials are also known as a negative trust reset™ within healthcare. Cost is a confusing issue. There are very few stakeholders that understand how money flows across the healthcare system. The U.S. health system is based on a "profit-maximizing approach" versus a relationship-based approach. (Khullar, 2020). This creates a foundation for the mistrust. In addition, the cost and financing structure of healthcare in the United States is fraught with myths. This creates challenges in understanding the impact of costs for each segment. These misperceptions have a negative impact on trust. Healthcare costs is one of those places where finger pointing is found and creates rifts in relationships and negative trust resets™ across the industry. Things such as increase in out-of-pocket costs to the healthcare consumer, the confusing and frustrating billing process for both providers and consumers, and the increasing costs of care to payers has fractured trust between stakeholders.

The issue of cost and its impact on trust is not a new issue. Payment models between patients and providers have changes over the last

50 years. With only a few exceptions such as the prepaid plans similar to Pierce County Medical Group and Kaiser Permanente, patients paid providers directly for the services that they received. This began to change in the 1980s. The increase of HMOs during that time brought the role of costs to the forefront. Many felt that decisions regarding care were often based on the cost of care and not the clinical appropriateness of care. Patients were not alone in this sentiment. Many providers also had concerns regarding the role that costs were playing in coverage decisions both in both the outpatient and inpatient setting. A study done in 1998 by Kao found that some of the newer payment models that included risk of monetary remuneration by providers created trust issues for patients. It was found that there were concerns that providers were not always acting in the patient's best interest. The survey found that patients that were receiving their care through the more traditional indemnity model were completely or mostly trusting their physicians to put their health and well-being about keeping the healthcare costs under control. The question remains almost 30 years later as to how healthcare should be financed, what is the correct pricing model, and who should be responsible in addressing cost issues within the healthcare system.

You cannot go through a week without the media speaking about the impact of healthcare costs on American consumers. During the 2020 Presidential election, healthcare costs have been considered the most important "dinner table" topic. A KFF survey found that two thirds of consumers are very worried and somewhat worried about being able to afford their own or a family members healthcare costs. (Pollitz,2020) Americans believe that in other countries people get their healthcare for free and that in the U.S. people have to pay. Although this is not the case, it creates a trust issue in the healthcare system as a whole.

Prior to the managed care era, there was little talk of cost impact on the consumer. Kao and his coauthors in 1998 found that over 75%

of patients surveyed completely or mostly trusted their physicians to "put their health and well- being above keeping down costs. (KAO 1998). This is no longer the case. As managed care plans insured more consumers, there was concern that the doctor was being "stingy" and was more concerned about cost to the health plan than in caring for the patient.

Over the last few years, there has been an increase in "financial toxicity" or the potential impact of cost of care for an individual and their family through the stresses that can be associated with cost of care. Studies have shown that between 44% and 64% of patients state that they have skipped care due to costs. (Healthcare Innovation). In addition, 13% stated that this deferral of care had negatively impacted their health. (Gupta, JAMA 2020). We found similar stories from our interviewees. Sam Glick, from Oliver Wyman, stated that consumers are paying a great deal of money with more of it coming out of their pockets and don't feel that they are getting value for this cost. This creates degradation of trust.

---

Increased Cost + Decreased value = Lack of trust

---

During the interview phase of our research, we asked people the following questions regarding healthcare finances

1. Is it your doctor's responsibility to take cost into consideration?
2. Do you believe that your doctor takes cost into consideration with your care and do you discuss costs?
3. Do you believe it is your responsibility to use cost as a determinant of what care to use and where to go for that care?

We found that each group of stakeholders within the healthcare ecosystem felt that others were responsible for high costs within healthcare. Doctors blame the hospitals, medical device, and pharmaceutical companies and even the patient for high costs. The pharmaceutical company executives blamed the insurance companies, the medical-legal system, the FDA, and other government entities. Insurance executives blame the patient, the doctor, the pharmaceutical companies, and the hospitals. A 2019 Kaiser Family Foundation analysis had similar findings to ours, consumers felt that the issue of cost blame was spread throughout the stakeholder environment including drug companies (78%), hospitals (71%), insurance companies (70%) and physicians (49%).

Although the patient looks to the doctor to focus on appropriate care, they also want the doctor to be conscious of what care is costing them. They want to discuss this with their doctors. Consumers are often willing to discuss costs but again, some are embarrassed that they cannot pay while others have a cultural dilemma in that it is their norm to separate financials from clinical interactions.

We asked the providers that we spoke with similar questions. They stated that they have difficulty in discussing costs for three reasons. First, providers stated that they are concerned that their patients will think that money is all that matters or that they will embarrass them. In addition, doctors are as unaware as the consumers when it comes to the cost of the care that they are suggesting. The third reason for not discussing the financial aspects of care is that they do not believe that there is anything that they can do to help.

Health Plans often take on the vitriol of the consumer for their perceived impact on consumer costs. We also had the opportunity to ask individuals a few financial questions about their health plans including; If you have a choice in health insurance companies, do you decide due to for profit status. Most of the people that were questioned during our survey admitted that they did not know whether their insurance company was a for profit or not for profit. A few believe that all health insurance plans were for profit. Most feel strongly that health plans should not be making a profit on the health concerns of others.

Consumers do not just focus on health plans in regard to the perceived injustice of healthcare costs. Pharmaceutical companies are also a focus of the frustration and distrust of consumers. Consumers see the high costs of their medications as disrespectful of them and cocky of the manufacturer. This anger has led to distrust.

> Thomas, a 41- year -old veteran, stated "no one should be making money off my illness. It doesn't not make sense. I go bankrupt trying to get better while the CEO of the insurance companies and the drug makers, makes millions of dollars."

Consumers are not the only ones that are frustrated about costs. Healthcare costs and the financial arrangements that underpin healthcare brings frustration to most of the stakeholders. It also tends to be a major negative trust reset™ across the entire industry. It is only over the last couple of decades that providers have spent any time focusing on costs. As far back as Aristotle's time, a portion of physicians did not accept payment. For many years, physicians would waive payments or took a reduced level of payment for their patients that were having trouble paying a bill. This was most commonly seen in cases where physicians owned their own practices. As the trend of providers being part of a large organization, this trend has receded. In fact, today it is not unusual for most providers to be disconnected from payments altogether. As providers became employees, their decisions associated with payment was removed. Many providers like this new model, as they believe that this allows them to focus on care and not cost. Unfortunately, this separation between care and cost has often created a trust challenge between the provider and the consumer. Providers are taught to render care to their patients based solely on science. They believe that they know what is best medically for the patient and that should be the focus not how much things cost. Costs to the patient or to society are not taught in medical school or in preparation for practicing medicine. Physicians admit that they often have little or no knowledge as to the cost of the care that they are rendering. (Carolyn Yao) (HIP 2018) Studies have shown that although many providers feel that discussing costs with their patients is important, few actually initiate a conversation regarding costs. (Annals of Internal Medicine, Vol 170, No. 9 May 2019) (Perez in his research found that less than 50% of those providers interviewed discussed out of pocket costs with their patients frequently.) A study from Rachael Greenup in J Oncology Practice, (Lowry)found that 80% of women who had been diagnosed with breast cancer had no financial conversation with their physician prior to making treatment decisions. Many of those questioned only initiated these conversations when they thought that cost may be impacting the outcomes of the care. We found during our interviews with patients and providers that most felt costs did play a role in a healthcare interaction but both sides were unclear as to how to initiate the conversation. In addition, many providers felt that they either little knowledge of what things cost, had few options as to how they could impact costs, or they felt they did not have the time to spend with their patient to talk about the issue. In addition, providers like to differentiate themselves from others within the healthcare environment. Providers often feel that health care executives including insurance executives, hospital executives and employers care more about costs then they do about the patient.

Dr Jones shared this story with me. She started out by saying that even though this happened over 25 years ago, it has greater impact today than it did at that time. Dr Jones treated a young patient of hers for an ear infection. This child had many ear infections over a short period of time and the medication that he most commonly used no longer worked. Dr Jones chose to use a new medication that had been very successful for a number of his patients. Later in that day, Dr Jones received a call from a pharmacy. The pharmacist stated that he had a patient's mother in front of him that had come to fill a prescription that he had written. She was quite angry and wanted to talk to me. She got on the phone and asked if I knew how expensive this medicine was. (I did not). She went on to say that I had embarrassed her because she could not afford the medicine. She asked me if I even cared about her and her child. Dr Jones spoke of her embarrassment and shared that she now always talks to her patients about cost.

Both consumers and providers commented on the issue of medications. It is important to understand that costs of medications, medical equipment and healthcare diagnostics have a far -reaching trust impact beyond just those two constituencies. In one study, 43% of individuals stated that cost concerns would keep them from getting the medicine and care that they needed. This was true regardless of age although millennials (61% would forgo care) were more cost sensitive than baby boomers (31% would forgo care). (WoltersKluwer,2020) Ian Reed, the CEO of Pfizer states that "in many ways, the pill is irrelevant. It is the knowledge needed to make the pill that really matters. We are the only ones that have this knowledge, and we should be paid for it". His comments were made on a national stage with stakeholders across the healthcare environment in attendance. The anger from the those in attendance was evident. A health plan executive turned to an employer and commented "this is why I never trust pharma". The good work of pharma manufacturers has been overlooked over the last decade due to the cost implications that have impacted the industry.

Cost issues also impact trust between employers, healthcare executives, hospitals, and the government. Most individuals know that their insurance coverage is through their employer but understand little more of their role in healthcare expenses. This has shielded the employer from the wrath of the patient over healthcare costs. That lack of knowledge does not pre-empt employers from being part of the cost conversation. Although cost issues are focused on insurance companies and pharmaceutical manufacturers, employers have a role to play. Employers, especially self -insured employers are ultimately responsible for the plan designs that are utilized and administered by the health insurance companies and pharmacy benefit managers. They have the power to choose the health plan and pharmacy plan that will cover their employees and their families. They also choose what is covered and the associated costs with care. The small portion of consumers that understand the decision -making role of the employer, either directly or indirectly, have articulated their frustration and anger over decisions such as facility fees, and rebate pricing of the medications that raise the consumer costs so that employers can receive rebate payments.

A new wrinkle in the cost and trust conundrum has arisen over the last few years, surprise billing. This billing and associated cost issue is example of the "blame game" that occurs in healthcare and creates a significant trust issue across the industry. Surprise billing is the unanticipated medical bills that arise when not expected by the consumer. The two most common causes of surprise billing are unexpected out of network charges from within an in-network system and facility charges that are not clearly articulated. A recent study found that 40% of those that utilized the emergency department of an in-network facility received a bill for out of network care, (Kaiser Family Foundation, 2020) and 18% of all in network hospital stays resulted in at least one out of network bill. An article by Sun and his co-authors found that surprise billing has continued to rise in both frequency and costs. This has not only increased distrust by the consumer but also by the government. The debate over unexpected charges has gained the increasing attention of Congress. The issue has arisen several times over the last few years. Late in 2020 a bipartisan group of Congress members agreed to a legislative fix to surprise billing. The bill if enacted would hold consumers harmless if the consumer cannot reasonably choose an in-network provider. The bill places the disagreement between providers and payers in the hands of a third- party dispute resolution system. The good news is that the consumer is out of the middle. Neither providers nor payers are happy with this solution.

Their very public disagreement has created distrust between the two groups. Throughout this debate, employers have remained silent .In addition, it has created a negative trust reset™ with consumers who feel that both groups are selfish and only focused on their own profits. This creates even further distrust.

Sally found that she was having increasing problems with her left knee. She had injured it years earlier in a snow skiing accident. As she has aged, the knee had become less stable and more painful. It had gotten to the point that the pain was keeping her up at night and she was having difficulty climbing her stairs at home. After conversations with both her primary care doctor and her orthopedist, it was decided that she would have a knee replacement. Sally did her research, she looked at all her options regarding costs and quality. She chose both a doctor and a hospital with high quality rankings that was in her network. The surgery went well, and Sally was recuperating and getting her life back to normal. Eight weeks after the surgery, Sally received a bill from the hospital for $32,000 for anesthesia services and for pathology. Sally's first reaction was that this must have been in error. After spending a significant amount of time on the phone with both her insurance company and the hospital, she found the answer to the issue. It was not an error. Although The anesthesiologist that sedated her and the pathologist that worked in the lab were located in the hospital that was in network, both providers were employed by independent organizations that did not have in network contracts with her insurance company. As Sally shared her story, her anger and frustration were palpable even after 3 years. Sally stated that these hidden fees impacted her trust not only on those that billed her but the doctors that cared for her, the hospital where she had the surgery and her insurance company that had told her which hospitals were in network. Sally stated that receiving this bill after trying to do the right thing, ruined her whole relationship with the healthcare system. "I do not trust it and will do everything I can to avoid engaging in the system."

Many of those that make financial decisions, do so without thinking about how the decisions impact on trust both within and outside of their stakeholder group. The lack of insight into this issue was consistent across all the stakeholder groups. It is time that decision makers add "trust impact assessments" to their decision matrix. (Jain S. JAMA, 2020)

Recommendations:

1. Individuals
   a. Don't be afraid or embarrassed to talk about costs.
   b. Create a systematic way in which to inquire into financial barriers to care for all patients. Don't do it just once but on a regular basis, either annually or when the health situation of an individual changes. Affordability is a keystone part of care.
   c. Consumers should understand their options and ask questions. Whenever possible, use cost tools that help you to understand the financial implications of your care decisions.
2. Organizations
   a. If a consumer cannot afford care, the best diagnostic, service, or treatment is worthless. Cost is everyone's issue
   b. Organizations need to redefine shareholder value in terms other than quarterly margin. This metric will eventually no longer be sustainable.
   c. Be aware that cost of care has a significant impact on trust. Don't make decisions regarding costs without understanding the long -term implications associated with the decision.
   d. Make the cost-trust impact assessment part of your decision matrix

   e.  If possible, have someone in the office that the provider can refer the patient to for help. This person should have the time and knowledge to understand potential options either within the healthcare system such as patient assistance programs or within the community.

   f.  When creating cost tools for providers and consumers, consider the following

      i.  Ability to personalize at the consumer level

     ii.  Ability to utilize at the point of care for both the provider and the consumer

## 8. Engagement

If we look back on the television show "Cheers". The group that was very diverse became the Cheers regulars because "everyone knew their name". Today the sense of community has been reduced and, in some cases, shredded. Engagement is an emotional connection. People want to interact with those that are open and friendly. They want to work with people that they like. Engagement is an important factor in gaining trust. Engagement builds loyalty along with trust. This is important for all the stakeholders within the healthcare environment.

Dr McEnery was a pediatrician in solo practice. He practiced at a time prior to electronic records and even paper medical records. His patient records were kept on 5x7 note cards. This was similar to most of his peers. Dr McEnery shared with me that the cards stored not only medical information on the patient but also important social information; Tommy trying out for soccer or Susan painting her room blue. This information allowed for "social cement™" and ways to engage the patient and their family the next time that they came into the office. It shows that you listen and that you care. The engagement level that Dr McEnery and his patients/families had created a trusted relationship that created better clinical outcomes. It also created a loyalty where this relationship lasted through two generations.

Engagement is not just the provider-consumer issue. Engagement is important throughout the healthcare environment both individually and organizationally. People work with people that they like. In addition, organizations that work to engage their employees, tend to have lower turnover. It makes work more fun. They trust the organization and the people that work with them. This builds motivation and long -term loyalty. Gallup's annual "State of the American Workplace" survey has shown that employee engagement increased not only profitability and employee retention, but also improved customer satisfaction.

Engagement is not always easy. It is not unusual for us to be time crunched or working under stressful situations. We live in a "check the box" world. We also are living within tight budgets. If something does not bring immediate value, we tend to dismiss it. Engagement is often one of those things that rarely is focused on and is often dropped.

Recommendations

1. Individuals
   a. Reveal yourself. Show vulnerability. A bit of social cement™ has been shown to improve engagement, relationships and trust. It also sets an example for an open engaging interaction. Authenticity verses power.
   b. Communication, both verbal and non-verbal help to build an engaged relationship with another person.
   c. Consider coming out to the waiting room and escort the others into the exam room or office. It equalizes power. This is a way to begin the engaged relationship. It is a few minutes well spent.

    d.   Identify "social cement" and document it so that you can remember it for future interactions.

2.  Organizations

    a.   Utilize organizational engagement surveys. This is not only important for the success of an organization internally, but it can also be used as an early warning sign of how your employees will treat others outside of the organization

    b.   Engage your employees. You can still separate personal and professional but engaging employees and helping them to feel "seen and known", has been found to be a valuable investment.

    c.   Employees that are engaged are more likely to be able to engage others, whether inside or outside the organization.

    d.   Utilize human centered design as the foundation that makes engagement easier

    e.   Prioritize connections and relationships over your products.

    f.   Build community within your organization. This magnifies engagement and brings greater value.

## 9. Experience-

Consumers expectations are higher than they have ever been. Historically, individuals expected reasonable quality and basic good manners. This is no longer the case. Recent changes in the retail experience have set a new standard for consumers. Consumer expectations do vary, depending on the individual and the setting. The one thing that does not vary is the need for being focused on the experience. Consumers do not delineate their expectations from one industry to another. Individuals do not consciously separate their lives into healthcare and non-healthcare. The experiences we have in our daily lives set the expectations and tone for what we expect within healthcare. The intensified consumer focus across other industries has increased the need for the healthcare industry to improve the experience. Think about going into a five -star hotel. The staff engages you immediately. They are friendly, helpful, take their time and ask you if there is anything else that they can do for you. You feel like you are the only person in the world. Let's also take a moment to consider the experience that Zappos offers. It is easy to order a pair of shoes online from Zappos. The company keeps you informed as to when your shoes will be delivered to you. It the shoes are not perfect, the return process is also quite simple. Why is one's experience working with others so important? Trust has been shown to be enhanced or eroded in each interaction. This is true whether we are talking about an individual's experience working with another person or with an organization.

An individual's experience is partially based on their expectations. Have you ever gone into a meeting expecting the experience to be horrible? Maybe the person that you are meeting with has a reputation of being mean spirited or the provider's office has a reputation for keeping people waiting for long periods of time. These beliefs create an expectation of what your experience will be. If the experience is expected to be poor and it is average, you may state that you have had a good experience. Whereas if the experience was good but expected to be great, one my find that the consumer evaluates the experience as average or poor. This is true both outside the healthcare environment as well as within the healthcare environment. Past experiences have a significant impact on trust. If the patients past experience is poor, it is likely that the patient will not trust the future experience and those involved. In the opposite, a good experience becomes a benchmark, and the patient is more trusting of the office and the doctor. Laura Holdsworth and her co-authors found that experiences that were deeply dissatisfying led to poor engagement and lack of trust in the relationship. She went on to find that the impact of these two factors lead to poor outcomes associated with the care received. There were three triggers associated with the dissatisfaction in the experience. They included system issues, technical processes, and interpersonal processes. Once someone is a victim of trust issues, they tend to trust less. We need to remember that regaining trust is not easy and is a journey. One thing that can help to rebuild trust, it is admitting that this poor past experience occurred.

Fukuyama in his 1996 paper wrote about trust "the expectation that arises within a community of regular, honest, and cooperative behavior, based on commonly shared norms, on the part of other members of that community". Whether it be an organization or the entire health-care ecosystem, we need to consider it a "community". A well -organized community works together for the community's best interest. This creates a trusting environment. As changes are occurring within the healthcare ecosystem, the shared historic norms, are changing. The institutionalization of healthcare has created an experience that creates distrust. We need to find ways to identify those norms that improve the experience and trust and then we need to better articulate those shared norms. Joe Babaian in a 2018 blog stated that trust in healthcare is based on experience, connections, and perception. Without this glue, the experience will erode any trust that we have within healthcare. Pierre Stephan, Accenture Engagement Practice Lead. "health systems need to provide effective, trusted, reliable care". This is important for both financial impact and potential long- term survival.

Accenture, in their annual survey found that patients feel like they have been "placed on the back burner". If their experience expectations are not met, it was found that they will switch providers including at the individual provider level, the hospital level, and the health system level. Experience leads to trust. Put simply, put patients first. This is true for not only patients, but for all individuals that are part of the healthcare environment. (Collado, 2017).

Not every experience goes as one would hope. It is important for providers of care, whether a pharmacy, a hospital or a doctor's office be aware of how processes are conducted and touch base with patients to see how their experience is perceived. One common mistake is to either formally or informally ask and then not take the feedback seriously. (Holdsworth, 2019)

> Dr. Manchine is an obstetrician that was well respected by both her patients and her peers. In speaking with her, she spoke of how important for everyone in the office to work towards a calm and caring atmosphere. This was important for both her patients but also the lives of their unborn children.

The Merriam-Webster dictionary describes a system as a set of principles and procedures to which something can be done. There are three attributes of a healthcare system that need to be considered when creating an experience that will have a positive impact on trust: organization, environment, and process.

**Organization-** In the past, healthcare was composed of the doctor, the patient and in some cases the insurance company. Over the last 30 years, the organizational model in healthcare has grown larger and more complex. Organizational models can be either a positive or negative trust reset™. Earlier we discussed the impact that new payment and organizational models associated with managed care in general and HMO in specific and how that impacted trust. Once again, we are in the midst of change. Roles of individuals are changing; payment and organizational models are changing. It is not just patients that are confused, many within the industry are confused as well. Confusion breeds both need of greater trust, but confusion also creates a decrease of trust. No one is quite sure of their roles and responsibilities. One Health Plan CEO we spoke to shared, "We are all bewildered. Many of the organizational structures that we have created in and of themselves create the degradation of trust, systems are not aligned, and value is often not reaped by those that are paying the largest amount for the services." This need for clarity becomes more important as we are realigning the relationship between providers and patients into a more aligned partnership.

The healthcare system is fragmented. This fragmentation creates not only confusion but difficulties in communication, collaboration, and alignment. It also creates a fracture in the continuity of care. Longer relationships create a stronger trusting bond. It is important to remember that consumers that trust their healthcare providers are more adherent to medicine, follow up more often and have better outcomes. In addition, a trusting relationship leads to higher satisfaction for both the provider and the consumer. Bilateral loyalty creates clinical and financial success for all parties involved.

Organizational issues can start badly and turn themselves around. Medicare Part D initially was poorly received. The program was overwhelming to consumers with choices that they did not understand and previously did not have to consider. In addition, there were a number of organizational problems and snafus. Over time both experience and fixes made Medicare part D a very popular and trusted healthcare option.

The impact of many of the organizational challenges that have occurred over the last 20 years is that of the healthcare silo. Consumers do not know who to rely on when they have a healthcare concern. Is it the employer benefits department, their health insurance carrier, their provider, the telehealth vendor, the urgent care center, or the emergency department at the local hospital? Adding to this complexity is the consumer that finds themselves in the hospital. The ill patient rarely sees their doctor, or provider they know and trust. Instead, they are cared for by a hospitalist that they do not know and that does not know them. At the time of discharge, there is once again confusion as to who is responsible for the care of the patient. What a mess. No wonder there is no trust. This organizational spaghetti bowl is built on competition and confusion. We must step outside traditional actions and activities toward a new integrated operating model if we want to regain trust between all stakeholders. Aligned incentives, better models of communication and the building of relationships are sorely needed.

**Environment**- Science has shown that the space around us can impact our behavior, our mood, and our productivity. The environment that we surround ourselves is a component of the non-verbal communication that articulates who we are. An orderly, clean, and welcoming atmosphere has been shown to lead to a mind -set that aligns with trust. It is important to consider who you will be interacting with. If there is a potential for you to be meeting with individuals with disabilities, make sure that your space is accommodating. This includes things such as color of the room, lighting, temperature, noise conditions and even whether there are indoor plants. "Good design is good business" Dan Greenfield the founder of Health Space Design. One's environment has been shown to increase collaboration and improve outcomes.

The environment such as office or hospital space plays a significant role within the clinical setting. Without consciously realizing it, healthcare consumers judge the healthcare that they will receive the moment that they walk into a provider office. Is the lighting warm and bright, is the furniture comfortable, the magazines up to date and the bathrooms clean? One study was done asking consumers about the furniture in their doctor's office. One consistent finding was that old furniture can create a feeling that you are lackadaisical and don't keep up with new care and treatment. Consider clean mid -range furnishings. You don't want to alienate someone with too high end or ragged old broken furniture.

Going to get medical care is never fun. Whether it is in a provider's office or a hospital, it is often anxiety provoking. In addition to indoor plants which have been found to be effective in both office and clinical facilities, fish tanks have been found to offer positive distractions for consumers waiting to receive care. They have been shown to reduce anxiety for consumers of all ages. In addition, diplomas on the wall are not bragging, they support the knowledge and the competency that the provider is looking to communicate to their patients.

Over the last few years, there has been an increase in the use of open workspaces. There is a belief that this type of internal architecture enhances collaboration. This may be true, but it also creates a challenge for those times where focus or privacy are paramount. This is especially important when personal health information will be shared. Offices and conference rooms should utilize round tables instead of the more traditional rectangular table shape allows for interaction without the inadvertent communication of power inequality. Computers and other technology should not be a barrier between individuals. It is very disconcerting when there is the perception that someone is multi-tasking or has distributed attention and not fully engaged.

**Processes**-How we interact with others is as important as who we interact with and where. First and foremost, the process should be as personalized as possible. Calling someone by their name shows that you are focused on them. A friendly demeanor goes a long way towards creating a positive encounter, reducing stress, anger, or the impact of bad news. Make things easy. As a consumer, making an appointment, to reach a provider with a concern or question, deciding what health insurance to choose, making things simple was important. Access and convenience are significant issues for all individuals. Difficulty navigating a system or getting an appointment creates issues of distrust. Romano and his team discovered that consumers had difficulties navigating health insurance plans and the healthcare system. The complicated system led these consumers to distrust both the plans themselves as well as the system as a whole. The providers that we spoke to also articulated their frustration with access to health plans. One provider shared his story about regularly being put on hold for 30 minutes or longer. Another talked about the insurance company's hours "not aligning with times that providers see their patients." It does not help when information or approval for the health plan is unavailable during office hours.

It has also been shown that access is not just an issue with health insurance plans, it is also a problem with providers. Many providers do not offer consumer centered hours. Are you there when I need you? 80% of individuals would switch providers for convenience. 50% said that access to care matters (NRC). In addition to access, rudeness impacts trust.

COVID 19 brought a new process issue to the forefront, that of physical safety. A recent Accenture study found that 25% of those surveyed stated that they did not feel safe when going to see a healthcare provider due to the pandemic. They felt that healthcare providers were either more concerned about their own safety or were not paying attention to the recommendations of the CDC. Those who did not feel "cared for" or "safe" stated that they "never plan to return or will at least wait." Sixty four percent were likely to switch health systems due to the company's lack of attention to safety and infection control.

Whether stated by healthcare providers or non-clinical healthcare workers, punctuality was a consistent frustration that led to a poor experience and a negative trust reset™. Edward G. Bulwer-Lytton said that "Punctuality is the stern virtue of successful men in business." This is true across healthcare as well, making the time to educate, communicate and build relationships is key. Everyone's time is important. Being on time and giving time shows respect. Individuals that are respected tend to trust those that respect them.

There are a number of new organizations that have reacted to the three attributes of a good experience and put them into action in the clinical setting. Provider organizations such as Oak Street Medical, Eden

Health, Zoom+ and One Medical have worked to create a welcoming environment, a consumer centric health care team, and an experience that creates a strong trusting bond between the team itself and the patients that they care for. Other organizations such as Quantum Health, Pager and Accolade have created an alternative support system for consumers in order to navigate and coordinate care. This helps consumers and their families to reduce the confusion and challenges to care.

1. Individual
   a. Put consumers or clients first.
   b. Don't assume that you are offering a positive experience. Only 51% of those survey felt that they had a good trusting experience and relationship with physician (Accenture 2020)
   c. Be on time. This means creating scheduling that works 90% of the time. For those times when you are running late, keep people notified.
   d. Don't overpromise and under-deliver. This creates a negative trust reset™ that is difficult to overcome
   e. Create a system that assures follow up on a timely basis.
2. Organizational
   a. Whenever possible utilize a human centered design approach. This methodology will help to contextualize both physical space and processes.
   b. Evaluate your physical environment, organizational structure, and processes to see if they create a positive or negative trust reset™. Review this on an annual basis along with input from others. Include internal and external customers in understanding expectations, creating, and operationalizing the experience. Utilize measurement tools such as Net promotor score (NPS). It has been long understood that satisfaction surveys are actually surveys measuring an individual's experience. (Baird, 2013). Types of qualitative feedback such as HCAHPS, NPS, or secret shopping

    c. Public disclosure of metrics and actions leading to improved outcomes should become a normal part of the annual reporting. Publicly traded companies should include this as part of the sustainability activities and should be rewarded for the positive trust reset™ that occurs with this activity.

    d. Create a physical space that creates a good experience and lends itself to a collaborative and trusting environment

    e. Utilize a personalized approach and experience. This increases engagement as well as leads to a greater likelihood of building trusting relationships

    f. Evaluate access points, either in person or telephonic. Make sure that access to support and appointments align with others needs and not just your own.

    g. Create a welcoming front door (both virtual and actual)

    h. Consider utilizing a secret shopper program in order to better understand the experience that others have with your organization.

## 10. Honesty, Integrity, and Ethics

As Friedrich Nietzsche stated, "I'm not upset that you lied to me, I'm upset that from now on I can't trust you." Honesty is an important factor in all relationships but especially important within healthcare. A person's health is one of the most personal aspects of their life and one where individuals are most vulnerable. It is an area where one person must rely on the knowledge and honesty of another in making life impacting decisions. We rely on the healthcare professional to place their needs behind that of the patient. William J. Bennett. The Author of The Book of Virtues stated that "To be honest is to be real, genuine, authentic and bona fide. Honesty expresses both self- respect and respect for others." Lance Secretan, an expert in Leadership also spoke about the challenges of honesty when he wrote that "We are suffering from Truth Decay." Studies confirm that one out of every five interactions between individuals includes a lie. (DePaulo, 1996) Sometimes it is an omission, in other cases it is considered a "white lie". Regardless, it is a situation where one person is not telling another person the truth. This lack of truth is a trust reset™ that can be difficult to overcome. Healthcare stakeholders need to actively address suspicion and distrust.

Where honesty is telling the truth, integrity means being honest in your actions, doing the "right thing in the right way". It shows that you have positive intentions and are acting in an honest manner, being true to your word, keeping your promises, and being dependable. Integrity is also having strong ethical principles that are followed regardless of the situation. Being honest and having integrity can be a challenge in healthcare. The ideal of beneficence is taught in most healthcare educational programs as we are trained to "do no harm" and to be honest and kind. Hippocrates, one of the most revered physicians in history stated that a doctor was the worst doctor in the world "if he does not promise to cure what is curable and to cure what is uncurable." (Katz) The question remains, is a physician lying if he states that he can cure something that is uncurable? Some people say that the truth can hurt, and that honesty is the best policy. What if a patient's health insurance does not cover the cost of a treatment, should the healthcare professional lie? We know that historically, doctors were not always honest with their patients. Early medicine was actually very opaque with the doctor having the knowledge and the patient trusting that the doctor would act in the patient's best interest without knowing much about the condition that they had or the treatment options. In fact, it was not until 1979 that most doctors were honest about a patient's cancer diagnosis. (Sisk 2016) Non-disclosure was the norm. This was considered the therapeutic privilege (Edwin AK, 2008) (Sisk, 2016) In fact, until the mid-20th century the AMA Code of Ethics stated that doctors should not reveal everything to their patients as it may endanger the health of the patient. This conscious non- disclosure within the Code of Ethics has long since been rescinded. Still today, there are certain cultures that do not believe that the dying should know their prognosis. That this information should either be withheld or that the patient be told a lie about their condition. The movie "The Ending" talks about the cultural norm within the Asian community to not be transparent with those that have terminal illness. In this movie, the female elder is suffering from cancer. The family does not want this information shared with her as they believe that it is their responsibility as the family to carry the burden of this difficult relationship. The movie talks about all the activity performed by the woman's doctor and her family to hide the diagnosis. In this case, the family would have lost trust in the physician if he had been transparent with the patient as to her diagnosis. What should a provider do if the family asks the provider to lie to the patient about their condition?

The question that is often not asked, is the patient meeting the expectation of the doctor? Are questions being answered honestly? Is the patient manipulating the doctor for gain such as in pain medication? Honesty and mutual trust bring value for all the parties involved. First, these qualities increase the likelihood of an improved outcome whether it be clinical or non-clinical. In addition, it is more fun and rewarding to work with those that you have a trusting and honest relationship with. The National Academy of Medicine has defined patient and family engaged care as "forthright, planned, delivered, managed and continuously improved in active trusting partnership with patients and their families." To achieve this goal, there needs to be honesty and trust on both sides. (Grob Racheal, Darien Gwen et al.) Simon Sinek reminds us that "being right does not make us trustworthy, being honest makes us trustworthy."

Healthcare is also one of the most regulated industries in America. Michael L. Michael, a senior fellow at the John F. Kennedy School of Government at Harvard University found that the more the regulated the industry, the greater the number of ethical misbehaviors. Healthcare is no different than other industries in that lapses in ethics are common. It is not unusual for us to see a headline regarding a stakeholder in healthcare acting in an unethical manner. One recent example is that of Purdue Pharmaceuticals. Their integrity has been lost due to the unethical marketing practices directly led to the oxycontin addiction issues that have confronted the country. This is a company that has lost trust across the healthcare industry. The Physician Payments Sunshine Act from 2010 was in reaction to another ethical challenge. The Act was due to the perceived and real issues associated with financial conflict of interest between pharmaceutical manufacturers and physicians or teaching hospitals.

We all make mistakes. Honesty about the mistakes we make is very important. Programs such as the Michigan Model for Medical Malpractice and Safety has taught us that honesty is the best policy. The process is counter-intuitive to the long- standing practice of withholding information on medical errors. This model utilizes early disclosure of error through communication with the patient, family and caregivers and fair compensation. This model has been shown to reduce malpractice claims and increase the trust between the providers, hospitals, patients, and the community at large. It is a great example of doing the right thing.

Honesty, integrity, and ethics all impact an individuals or organizations reputation. The Edelman 2020 Trust Barometer found that reputation and ethics are three times more important in building trust than most other factors. Another recent study found that 39% of those surveyed feels that brand reputation is the most important factor in trust. (NRC).

Honesty and integrity lead can build or destroy one's reputation. One challenge is when one stakeholder has a good reputation but is associated with others with a poor reputation. This can create a negative trust reset ™ and impact an organization's trust impact scores.

1. Individual
   a. Be self-aware, accountable, responsible, truthful, and consistent.
   b. Be yourself
   c. Do what you say you will do
   d. Honesty is not always easy. Healthcare has rules that do not always make sense and are not in all stakeholder's best interest. You may be inclined to be dishonest to reach the desired goal or outcome. Do not give in to that desire as it will often lead to a negative trust reset™ , even if you have good intentions. The end does not justify the means.
2. Organizations
   a. The honest and ethical behavior of the leadership of an organization will impact the employees and the organization as a whole. Honesty, ethics, and integrity are components of good governance.
   b. Understand the organizations morals. What do you stand for? Be honest with yourself. If you say that you are looking to help an individual, do your actions reflect your words? If they do not, you will not be perceived as honest and others will not trust your words or your actions.
   c. Keep your agreements
   d. Keep company with honest and high integrity organizations. You are reflected by the company that you keep

## 11. Incentives-

Our behavior as humans is based on the incentive theory of motivation. We are inspired by the desire to gain reinforcement such as incentives. Humans are predictable. In most cases we will follow our own self interests. This shapes our behavior. Aligned goals and incentives are an important factor in creating and maintaining trust. There is risk to trust. The risk is that one party will take advantage of the trust that the other has given them in order to benefit themselves. Misaligned or competing incentives can create competition and even hostility. Motive has an important role in trust. If one does not understand the motive of another, it becomes difficult to trust. Clear and recognized motives can either be an enhancer or destroyer of trust. One needs to refrain from assuming a motive as that assumption is often incorrect. Transparency of motive for all parties decreases assumptions and allows for open discourse that can frequency lead to the beginnings of trust. Individuals, whether a consumer, provider, healthcare executive or government or policy person, all want to know that their best interests are being considered.

Fraud, abuse, and waste in the U.S. health system costs us over 760 billion dollars. (Shrank et al. 2019). Much of this is due to misaligned goals within the system. Physicians and hospitals have been paid for services given versus the outcomes of those services, medication formularies are created through contractual agreements that are incentivized through drug rebates and other forms of payments, and some health insurance brokers are paid to recommend one insurance company over another. None of these incentives focus on the outcome of effective medical care. What if the value -based contracts brought direct value to not only consumers but payers and providers as well?

Incentives are not only money based, in some cases it is reputation or power based. The United States government is a good example of this. When the government supports, passes, or blocks the passage of a law, it shows their power. Their incentive has little to do with the purpose of the law. The passage of the Medicare Modernization Act of 2003 which put Medicare Part D in place and the Affordable Care Act of 2010 are two examples of this. In each case, one party strongly approved of the laws and the other strongly disapproved. Much of the disagreement was political. Health care policy is often used as a political weapon with power being the incentive. What if all members of the government had to live with the implications of these laws? If the incentives of the consumer and the government were aligned, we would likely have a different outcome.

We do have a challenge, those who are responsible for control and payment are not always the stakeholder that receives value and is most impacted. In order to align incentives, we have to agree on a goal and then bring all stakeholders to the table to be represented. Only then can we use incentives as a positive trust reset™ tool.

Recommendations

1. Individual
   1. Be open and willing to acknowledge the incentives that you are basing your actions on.
   2. Identify areas in which your incentives are aligned with others
   3. Understand that in most power based incentive struggles, neither side really wins. If possible, find incentives and goals that you can agree with and remove barriers to success
2. Organizational
   1. Be aware that incentives can be based on financials or power.
   2. Today's healthcare structure is based on action versus outcome. Begin to find ways to transform that structure
   3. Partnering instead of competition can lead to greater alignment in incentives
   4. Creation of cross-stakeholder performance measurements and contractual arrangements associated with those measures in order to align end purpose goals. When all stakeholders are not considered, negative trust resets™ are likely to occur.
   5. Creation of infrastructure to successfully achieve the aligned measures
   6. Be willing to disclose incentive structures with all stakeholders. The specifics, when appropriate, can still remain private.

## 12. Privacy and Confidentiality-

Confidentiality has been an issue as far back as Hippocrates. The Hippocratic Oath states, "I will not divulge, as reckoning that all such should be kept secret". Years later, the AMA Code of Ethics makes similar statements by devoting significant attention to the issue of privacy and confidentiality., "Patients need to be able to trust that physicians will protect information that is shared in confidence". History has been a major tenant and consistent in its point of view that health care providers should not discuss a person's healthcare with another individual without the patient's permission. There are a few instances when confidentiality can be breached. Confidential information can be shared by a healthcare provider when the patient themselves or another individual is in "clear or imminent danger". The AMA Code of Ethics does articulate this formally and state that authorities should be notified under these circumstances and if child abuse or neglect is believed to be occurring. A third area where confidentiality laws can be breached is when it can impact public health. Laws such as the Human Rights Act of 1998 discusses the "respect for private life" but also includes clauses that discuss this right being overridden for the "protection of the public health". (O'Brien, 2003). This exception to confidentiality has come into play several times in the last fifty years including during the AIDS crisis in the 1980s and during the COVID crisis of 2020. These exceptions have created concerns from consumers and have been shown to impact their willingness to seek care and share personal health information.

Privacy is the "right of an individual to be let alone and to make decisions about how personal information is shared." (Brodnick, 2012). Public areas in clinical settings and public spaces outside of clinical settings all create risks of information being shared without approval. In today's fast pace and mobile world, it is easy to forget about the need for privacy.

George was getting on an elevator in the building where one of his doctors had his office. In the elevator were three people in scrubs. George found himself in the middle of the conversation of the three who were talking and laughing about a patient. The elevator opened and George as well as the other three got off the elevator. George then walked into his doctor's office. To his surprise and dismay, George found that the three people that he shared the elevator with were staff in his doctor's office. George shared with us during his interview that he never felt comfortable sharing all his intimate information with his doctor or nurses because he could not trust that it would be treated as confidential.

Dr. Drago is a family physician that tells the story of his being in a restaurant with his family and receiving a call from a patient. He did not want to interrupt the family dinner, so he took the call at the table. At the end of the call, a gentleman from the next table walked up to him and let him know that he had heard every work that Dr. Drago had said. The gentleman went on to say how unprofessional it was and that he would make sure that his friends did not seek care from Dr. Drago. Dr. Drago learned his lesson

The issue of confidentiality for a consumer is tied to trust. If you are concerned that your information will be shared, you are less likely to be open and honest. When providers do not respect their patient's privacy, the patient feels that the provider is "not on their side and does not have their back". This is especially true with certain conditions that have stigma associated with them such as HIV/AIDS, sexually transmitted conditions, drug and alcohol abuse and other mental illness. Consumers consistently articulate their concern that public knowledge about their health can have financial, healthcare coverage and job consequences if shared. Although the Affordable Care Act mandated that pre-existing conditions could not impact health care coverage or premium costs, consumers still do not trust the health-care insurance industry with their medical history. They also are wary of trusting employers with this information as they believe this information may have potential impact on their employment status.

Confidentiality exists in healthcare outside of the consumer and provider relationship. Business and contractual agreements between stakeholders also are subject to both legal and ethical confidentiality rules.

> Joellene, is a senior executive for a hospital system. She was on a flight sitting next to two gentlemen that were discussing a contract that had just been signed. Joellene, laughed as she shared this story. She shared with me that the contract that was signed was with a competitor. She overheard a great deal of private competitive information that she should not have heard. It reminded her that there are "ears" everywhere.

The confidentiality issues around these types of business interactions received much attention over the last few years. Financial and business agreements between providers, insurance companies, pharmacy benefit managers, pharmaceutical manufacturers and others impact the cost of and access to care. There has been dialogue, court cases and most recently legislative action focused on whether these arrangements should remain confidential. This conversation has created negative trust resets™ in a number of ways. Consumers do not trust the other stakeholders as they do not understand why they need to be kept confidential, while the stakeholders that are part of the agreements are concerned over the impact of these arrangements losing confidentiality. The final decision on this and its impact is yet to be seen.

Issues associated with data privacy have become even more central recently. The amount and type of health information has increased over the last decade. The increased use of connected devices, remote monitoring, and new forms of communication, have all created informational "fumes" that are at risk of being shared inappropriately. In addition, there has been an increase in organizations using data for purposes outside of the original intent. Data sales across stakeholders has become common place. In many cases, those whose data is being sold is unaware that this activity has been occurring. As this endeavor has reached the national consciousness, it has created a negative trust reset™ around an individual sharing their data and has created greater focus on information privacy. The Heath Insurance Portability and Accountability Act (HIPAA) Privacy Rules were put in place in 2006, to create a national standard for privacy protections associated with an individual's healthcare protected information. The rules had three areas of focus including administrative, physical, and technical measures necessary to protect healthcare data. Once again, like other laws associated with privacy and confidentiality, there are exceptions. Regardless, the impact of data privacy breaches is far-reaching and can impact the trust that others have in the organization and its reputation for years to come. It will also impact healthcare's ability to innovate and move forward scientifically.

Recommendations

1. Individual
   a. Understand patient confidentiality laws. Do not rely on others such as office staff to take responsibility. This includes the rules around "minimal necessary" information obligations.
   b. Discuss privacy and confidentiality rules with your patients and their families. This will help them to understand the importance that you place on the issue. Make sure that you ask consumers who they would like to be included in conversations and decision making.
   c. Document all appropriate requests of patients requests to share their information. Include all signed documentation pertaining to information sharing in the patient records

d.  Make sure that all paper documentation is safely kept in locked cabinets when not in use. Do not take these documents out of the office.
e.  Make sure that all electronic health information has the appropriate safeguards.
f.  Do not have private conversations with others where they can be heard by third parties, this includes in hallways, elevators and nursing or workstations, and other public places such as restaurants.

2.  Organizational
    a.  Create a privacy and security culture for all forms of information
    b.  Create policies and confidentiality agreements for both internal and external stakeholders
    c.  Provide training for all employees and contractors
    d.  Utilize both blockchain and encryption tools for all healthcare data.
    e.  Language interpretation has become an increased area of need for many healthcare organizations. It is also an area of confidentiality and privacy risk. Make sure that there are processes and training in place when language interpretation is being utilized.
    f.  Perform regular assessments of health information risks
    g.  Create protection for all medical information whether it be written or electronic
    h.  Make sure that there are areas available for private conversations. This is necessary in both clinical and non-clinical areas. Place visual reminders in areas of high risk about private conversations.

## 13. Respect

Aretha Franklin sang a well- known adaption of Otis Redding's song R-E-S-P-E-C-T. The chorus says, "find out what it means to me." This acknowledges that there is no single definition of respect, just as there is no one definition of trust. When we asked consumers what it means for them to be respected by their healthcare providers, we heard words such as caring, empathetic, dignity, recognition and individual or autonomous.

> Steven, a 33- year- old male said "I expect my doctor to check his ego at the door. I look for him to see me as an individual, important in the relationship and equal in importance to him. This is how he shows me respect. It is also how I will gain respect for him."

The definition of respect is to consider another individual worthy of esteem. There are some individuals that believe that they should be respected due to their educational level, title, role, or demographics. This is not the case. Respect is earned by one's actions and not by other attributes. Actions that gain respect include doing what you say you are going to do, being useful, bringing value to the relationship, being humble and bringing humility to your actions and successes. In addition to actions that can positively impact respect and trust, there are things that you should not do such as making excuses, taking credit for others work or gossiping.

Respect is an important ingredient to the creation of relationships. It is hard to have a relationship with someone that you do not respect. Gaines talks about the social psychological aspect of respect; the "social acceptance of another person". This seems to align with other views of respect, including that of those that we spoke to. (Frosch, 2014) The United States is a multi-cultural country. How people choose to be addressed or what they consider appropriate amounts of personal space vary by culture and demographics. What you call someone is a form of respect. In many Asian culture names are listed in a different order, in other cultures it is inappropriate to call someone by their first name unless invited to do so. It is important that an individual is called by their preferred name and that name is correctly pronounced. It means that you are "seen" and "known". As Dr Richard Baron, the President and CEO of the American Board of Internal Medicine Foundation has stated, this is the "axis of a relationship" as it shows respect.

The healthcare system should be based on relationships. Unfortunately, today it is based on hierarchy. Historically, healthcare was based on a paternalistic model of relationship. Physicians assumed and received respect due to their education and title.

> Ethel has been a practicing nurse for 20 years and her mother is a nurse. She is a middle aged African American woman. She has had the same physician for almost 20 years. She likes her physician but does not totally trust him. "We were brought up to be wary of our healthcare providers. We don't feel totally safe that they have our best interest in mind and not have ulterior motives." She goes on to share that the experience of the Tuskegee syphilis experiment is always back of mind. "I am not sure if he does not respect me because I am a woman, a black person or because I am not a doctor and do not have the same education as he does."

Patients that perceive that they are disrespected by their doctors are less likely to trust both that provider as well as the information and advice that they are given. Thirty five percent of lower income privately insured individuals feel disrespected by providers. These people are three times more likely not to believe their doctors compared with those that do feel respect. (Oliver Wyman, "Right Place, Right Time: Improving access for healthcare information to Vulnerable Patients) (A Matter of Trust, Modern Healthcare June 24, 2019 pp 24).

As consumerism has grown to be a more prevalent part of healthcare, the model is changing. Activities such as shared decision making requires a more equal relationship with mutual respect between the consumer and the provider. Hierarchy is common across health-care; between specialists, hierarchy within healthcare between different types of clinicians (pharmacists, nurses, and doctors), between healthcare specialties, between business healthcare executives and doctors, and between doctors and patients. Whether this is a power issue, or a knowledge issue is not always clear.

The mutual respect between providers and consumers is not the only area within healthcare shown to be an important factor in creating successful organizations and relationships. Individuals whether providers, payers, patients, or policy makers all need to respect each other if we are going to regain trust. Success requires people to focus on what is important instead of participating in a power tug of war. Collaboration and reciprocity increase trust where power plays, coercion and other forms of pressure decrease trust. This is not the behavior that we see today. It is not unusual for doctors to assume that they are the "top" of the hierarchy and demand respect from other health-care providers, whether they be doctors, nurses, pharmacists, social workers, or the many other healthcare providers that are part of the healthcare team. It is also not unusual for the non-clinical healthcare workers to work in a competitive, win-lose position versus in a mutual respectful environment. Non-clinical individuals often disrespect the knowledge that that clinicians bring, while clinical professionals disrespect the decisions that non-clinical professional have to make, stating that they do not care about patients. The ability to give honest feedback without the fear of reprisal is crucial.

Why does respect increase trust? For patients, respect often equates to psychological safety. Safety has been found to have a significant impact on the provider and consumer relationship. Healthcare involves vulnerability. Trust is often defined as " a psychological state comprising the intention to accept vulnerability based upon positive intentions or behavior of another in creating a safe environment" (Academic Medicine, June 2019). Many of those we spoke to talked about their vulnerability. **Vulnerability requires a trusting relationship for "survival"** . Showing vulnerability allows for a "safe space" for trust to grow in a mutual manner. Trust is one of the things that helps us to overcome our fears and vulnerability when it comes to trust. A shared vulnerability and experience lead to trust "they know what I am going through" . Eric Cassells, MD said "sick people are people who are forced to trust". You may ask, why do they need to trust? It is due to their vulnerable state.

> Rachelle is a 70-year-old woman. Until recently she has been quite healthy. Unfortunately, Rachelle fell and broke her hip. She called her son who was a doctor to come and be with her in the hospital. During her stay, she had become quite frustrated as she needed help to get up from the bed and therefore had to buzz for hospital staff to come and help her to get up. Unfortunately, staff was not always able to get there in a timely basis. Her son wanted to discuss this with his mother's care team in the hospital. Rachelle shared with me her fear of this conversation occurring. She was fearful that the team would be mad and then not take care of her. Her vulnerability placed her in a place where she did not feel safe from repercussions.

Respect also impacts the non-clinical environment in healthcare. People that feel respected are more likely to feel included, bring their best game and therefore be more productive. Feeling respected allows someone to feel safe and trust that the other person or the organization has their back.

> Delwin was an executive within a Pharmacy Benefit Management company. The CEO called a meeting of the executive team. During the meeting, one of the attendees asked the CEO about one of the new policies that was being put in place and the reasoning behind it. The CEO took a deep

breath and then stated that it was an executive decision and that the team should just obey his orders. He then went on to ask if there were any other questions. Delwin stated that the room became silent due to the lack of safety the team felt in asking any other questions and the lack of respect that the CEO showed his executive team.

If an individual does not feel respected, they may feel that they were not safe in their job and can be easily replaced. This in turn creates dissatisfaction and distrust among individuals. Not feeling respect can also undermine one's confidence. This can create a less then optimal outcome at a time when all stakeholders have to be at the top of their game. In recognition of the importance of respect within an organization, Virginia Mason launched a "Respect for People" initiative in 2012. Their program supported the identification of the importance of respect between all employees and then put in place educational programs so employees could respect and appreciate their co-workers.

Recommendations

1. Individual
   a. Don't assume that you will receive respect automatically due to title, job, or demographics. Respect, similar to trust should not be assumed.
   b. Power playing, bullying, or degrading others does not create respect.
   c. Identify those areas that show respect such as values, cultural differences, and knowledge.
   d. Do not act in ways that reduce respect such as making excuses for poor outcomes, taking credit for other's actions or successes, gossiping, or speaking badly about others. People do not respect this as they are concerned that you will do this to them.

2. Organizational
   a. Mutual respect begins at the top. Leaders should set the expectation of respect.
   b. Identify and recognize those actions that build respect. Create educational and support programs that create respectful interactions.
   c. Discourage those actions that can negatively impact respect. Document incidents and provide feedback when these actions occur regardless of who the individual is.

## 14. Technology

Technology has become an important tool, integrated into most American's lives. Pew research found that 40% of Americans feel that technology has improved their lives over the last 50 years and will continue to do so. Twenty percent state that the biggest improvement will be in the areas of medicine and healthcare. (Pew Research Center, 2016). The impact of technology on healthcare has been increasing for the last forty years. The use of technology has spread across the healthcare domain through the internet for information, electronic health records and portals for documentation and communication, virtual care including remote monitoring between providers and consumers, tools for diagnosis and treatment, consumer technology for the quantified self and communication between healthcare stakeholders. Technology has been both a positive and negative trust reset™ for consumers and the industry. There has been quite a bit of conversation as to whether the increased use of technology impacts the trust in a relationship. Part of this depends on whether the technology is replacing the human elements that normally bind the two stakeholders. Consumers trust in technology is multifaceted.

The impact of technology on healthcare is not a new conversation. In 1816, a new health technology was introduced. There was great concern that this new technology would come between the consumer and the provider and that it would impact the trust between the two individuals. This technology was a stethoscope. There was great concern that the stethoscope replaced a conversation between the consumer and their physician about their symptoms. (Heath, 2018). Fast forward to 2020 and technologies impact on trust within healthcare.

The availability of the internet has had an impact on both consumers and providers. Healthcare information easily accessed via the internet is a great equalizer when it comes to basic healthcare information. The "informatization" (Seckin, 2014) has created a "democratization" of healthcare. This capability has impacted the paternalistic nature of healthcare by allowing consumers to be more active participants in their health and healthcare. It also allows providers up to date information on the newest aspects of healthcare. The internet created democratizaion of information that can both positively and negatively effect trust between the provider and the consumer. The impact depends on issues such as:

1.  How do consumers decide on which internet sites to trust as they look for information?
2.  How consumers and providers respond to those instances where the information that they find on the internet is in conflict with what their doctor has said.

Early in the history of internet availability, while I was still practicing medicine, I had a patient with a child that had uncontrolled asthma. I suggested to this mother that we try steroids on her son to see if we could control his asthma. This young man's mother was very concerned about steroids due to her confusion, and apparently my inability to help clarify, that these steroids were different from the steroids that caused numerous side effects such as violence that she heard discussed in the news. She asked to have a few days to think about it. I told her that this was fine. I gave her some information to read and helped her to make an appointment the following week. At the follow-up appointment, the mother handed me over 100 pages from the internet that she had printed out. The information that she had read and then given me were from a variety of internet sites, many of them with little connection to evidence -based science. She wanted to know why I was not trying any of the things that were described in the information that she had given me. It took us several weeks to sort things out and for her to understand the different levels of information that were available to her. It took six weeks, but we were eventually able to get to an agreement that we would try her son on inhaled steroids. I do not believe that we would have gotten to that conclusion if we did not have the relationship and mutual trust that came from it. Her son did so well on his inhaled steroids that he received a 100% attendance the next school year after missing numerous days in the past. I also learned an important lesson about proactively addressing the internet and identifying sites that provide legitimate information.

Unlike my experience, a 2014 study found that almost 50% of consumers that use the internet to research information rarely or never discussed that information with the provider because of concerns about how their providers would react to their research. Of those that did discuss their research with their providers a large portion stated that this conversation helped to strengthen the relationship with their providers. (Seckin, 2014)

Providers do have an opinion on their patients who do their own research. A 2009 article defines a condition called Cyberchondria. This condition occurs when consumers self- diagnose with the information that they find on the internet. In addition, providers speak about their concern regarding reliability of the information that they find, and concern over the time it takes to discuss the information brought to the visit. Acceptance of consumer -initiated research has increased over the last 13 years. Many providers have found that this activity has increased consumer engagement and improved trust between the provider and the consumer.

Similar to the use of the internet by consumers and providers, electronic medical records and portals have had a both positive and negative impact. This form of technology allows healthcare providers to access their patient's data from anywhere. This improves the experience and outcomes that a consumer has with their medical providers. On the other hand, there has been frustration articulated by both providers and consumers as to the negative impact on the relationship. The EMR has often been considered the barrier to the provider and consumer interaction due to challenges in eye contact, non-verbal communications, and lack of real time interaction. "There is always this wall between my doctor and I" is a comment we heard a number of times.

Consumer portals connected to electronic medical records can help ease the transactional activities that occur within healthcare. Activities such as making an appointment, refilling medications, accessing health data, billing information, and paying bills. How individuals communicate has changed over the last forty years. Historically, healthcare communication in healthcare has occurred via face to face, telephonic and beepers. The era of beeper is over. Today, the consumer portal can improve communication in a more effective and efficient fashion. Providers and consumers can communicate in an asynchronous manner at a time that is good for both. This creates a trusting relationship because the consumer knows that they can communicate with their provider. In addition, the conversation is documented for both parties. This makes it easier to go back and look at past conversations and/or continue the conversations at a different time. That being said, there is a great deal of frustration around the use of the portal for some interactions. Many consumers felt that the portal is used as a gatekeeper for conversations that they feel are important. "This puts the doctor in total control of how and when I interact with them. Have you ever tried to have a follow up conversation with your doctor? Near impossible. They call back when it is convenient to them. They don't ask when you are available. At least in the old days, my doctor had call in hours."

In addition to the patient portal as a communication conduit, virtual care and monitoring has taken on a more significant role in the relationship between consumers and providers. The use of technology tools has increased over the last few years. COVID 19 has expanded the usage of virtual or telehealth considerably. For a large portion of 2020, the only way for individuals to receive care outside of the emergency department was through technology. It is unclear what the utilization trends will be as the pandemic is controlled and life returns to a more normal cadence. It is clear that many providers and consumers have come to trust virtual visits over the last year. This has been especially true in the case of mental health support. This is not true for everyone. Issues still exist for a portion of the population, privacy, worry that the provider may be multi-tasking and the creation of a trusting relationship have been cited as concerns. In addition to increases in telehealth utilization, COVID 19 has increased the use of remote monitoring health markers such as blood sugar, blood pressure, weight, and heart rate. A 2018 Oliver Wyman survey found that 42% of respondents trust their physicians to monitor their health condition through wearable technology. As you notice, the individuals stated that the trust came from the fact that it was their primary care provider that was engaged in the monitoring. A relationship already existed. As discussed, trust is most often found in an existing have already formed relationship.

There are presently approximately 266 million smart phone users in the United States. (Statistica.com, April 2020) This equates to 96% of Americans. Over 50% of these individuals have at least one app downloaded on their phone with on average 7 being health or healthcare related. When you realize that there are over 47,000 healthcare apps available, there is actually a small number being downloaded and utilized. These apps offer health related services to the consumer providing information across the healthcare and health spectrum. They allow the consumer to engage in their health in a mobile manner matching their lifestyle. These apps can help to communicate with their providers, their caretakers, or other consumers. They monitor health and disease, share real time data about their issues with providers and help them choose the best course of action in managing their own conditions. Most individuals do not know who actually created the app, what information was used to create the app and how the information will be stored and used by others than the consumer and the provider. Trust tends to be stronger if the technology is suggested or provided by the providers that the consumer trusts. Trust breeds trust. Overall, consumers trust health apps more than other technology tools utilized in healthcare. Our research found that 43% of those that we surveyed were using a health app to track their progress. One reason for this is a perception that they have control over the apps and the information that is created within the app. If there is distrust or they don't bring value, they can delete them.

Technology is not only utilized by providers and consumers and hospitals. Since the onset of COVID 19, technology is been the cornerstone of most of our lives. We have learned to trust technology in order to interact and stay in touch with family, friends and colleagues. We have shopped, been entertained, be educated, run organizations, be engaged, and loved through the use of technology. All of us, including the stakeholders involved with healthcare, have relied on technology to communicate, and do that what has to be done.

Technology is a valuable trusted tool if understood and used correctly. When technology is integrated into an existing relationship, it has been shown to have a greater liklihood of strengthening trust. The pandemic created a timeline for the use of technology that was placed on hyperdrive. One healthcare executive stated "it is amazing what you can do when you have to. We fast forwarded technology but at least five years. We had no choice. We had patients to care for". Cheryl Pegus MD, past President of Consumer Health Solutions and Chief Medical Officer of Cambia and now EVP of Health and Wellness for Walmart recently articulated the challenge associated with technology and trust; "people's relationship with technology can be complicated, much like health care's relationship with the technology industry as a whole. People seek conveniently assessable and definitive answers, while reserving a certain amount of trust in a human connection". None the less, almost 75% of consumers say that they are willing to change providers in order to assess telehealth care. While they understand access and convenience, a 2017 study found that more than 50% of consumers have concerns and trust issues about the benefits of health care information technology. Many of the concerns have to do with privacy. There is concern that the information acquired by technology will be given to employers or government without their consent. Digital and data breaches continue to have a negative impact on trust. This includes trust in the technology, as well as trust in those that suggested the use of the technology

Technology as "the" tool is not a replacement for the interactions and relationships that positively impact relationships. There are a number of instances where technology just cannot work. Issues such as broadband and digital competence are very real factors when looking at experiential and outcomes. As Kara Trott, the Founder and CEO of Quantum Health said, "Technology cannot hug you when you are confused and scared". None the less, technology can be effective if use in the right way and at the right time. Technology can improve access of care and cost of care for the consumer. It can improve effectiveness and efficiency for the provider. It can improve engagement and outcomes for employers, and health plans who are payers of the care.

Assumptions cannot be made. The use of technology must be done diligently and thoughtfully. Concerns exist and have to be addressed.

Major concerns include legal issues, payment issues, operational issues and most importantly, how relationships are impacted. High touch integrated with technology can allow for increased support and engagement.

Recommendations

1. Individual
   a. In most cases, technology should not replace the foundational interactions between two individuals. This is true for all relationships within healthcare. Use of technology for transactional purposes, can actually support time and energy for the "intimate moment of healthcare" in a high touch manner.
   b. Providers should proactively discuss the use of the internet and healthcare apps for their patients and give their patients a recommended list of resources that they trust.
   c. Providers should pro-actively discuss the use of the electronic medical record. Share your desire to have an authentic relationship with your patients. When possible interact at least part of the time away from the computer.
   d. Technology can enhance workflow if done correctly. Understand your workflow and where technology enhances workflow. Remain focused on the impact on others.
2. Organization
   a. Evaluate the strengths and weakness in the use of technology. Utilize customer- centric design tenets to help address the weaknesses and magnify strengths of technology. This helps to understand the role and the value of healthcare technology and how to appropriately use it. Understand that technology for the sake of an organization may not give the desired goals if the value is focused on the organization and not the users. This creates both negative trust resets™ but also commoditizes the experience.

b.  When possible, initiate important relationships through face -to -face interactions. This builds the basis for a long -term, trusted relationship. This will allow for the successful use of technology for many further interactions.

c.  Base payment models for the use of technology in the healthcare environment on value. This removes the win-loss and payment for activity challenges in healthcare.

d.  Privacy and security are important factors in whether technology is a positive or negative trust reset™ . Create clear and regular assessments of security standards. Articulate those to all stakeholders that the organization interacts.

e.  Clearly articulate how the data "fumes" associated with technology will be utilized. Understand the tradeoffs of sharing data with third parties for financial gain.

f.  Understand that if technology does not support the building of relationships and trust, it is hurting it. Technology needs to build humanity and not replace it.

## 15. Transparency

Merriam-Webster dictionary defines the word transparency as "much is known by many" and "the process of being open and honest." There are some individuals that believe honesty and transparency are the same action. The words are connected but not the same. Honesty is when one person tells another person the truth. Transparency is the act of making information known so that a person can decide the truth. Both actions can be associated with a positive or negative trust reset™. Bridget O'Brien in a 2019 article spoke of the impact of transparency in society as having this result: "Public trust in institutions and peoples trust in one another would run high because all information worth viewing is readily available." (O'Brien, 2019). She spoke of the "transmission of information" that is accurate, objective, and comprehensive. Unequal access to accurate information creates "mistrust, inefficiency, skepticism and various other problems" (O'Brien, 2019). The common theme heard during our conversation was associated with the belief that information is power. There are many individuals that feel that the lack of transparency in healthcare is done on purpose as a means of hiding information. Over the last 30 years the issue of transparency has increased in focus within the healthcare environment. It has become a "poster child" in causes for distrust across the industry. The conversations have varied depending on the stakeholder group. Consumers have focused their comments on issues such as healthcare costs or quality. Providers concentrated on the barriers to transparency while health care executives talked about it in terms of colleagues withholding information in order to gain "the upper hand". These conversations demonstrate how a lack of transparency can be a trust buster while its presence can create a positive and trusting relationship.

Costs have taken center stage over the last 10 years as payers, including employers, health plans, and governmental agencies look to address the unsustainable increase in healthcare costs. One of the levers that is being used to address this is the increasing focus on changing the "patient paradigm" to a "consumer paradigm". We have asked individuals to treat healthcare in a similar fashion as other goods and services that they purchase. For the most part, a consumer's daily interactions are transactional. "I will give you this, if you give me that". The rules are set, and the exchange happens (or not).

> Valerie was looking to hire a new individual to clean her home. She interviewed the person and then asked what cleaning her home would cost. The person stated that she did not know and would not know until she cleaned the house a number of times. Valerie asked for a range of what this person charges others who houses she cleans. The individual stated that she would not share this. On the surface, not knowing how long the cleaning would take and therefore how much it would cost makes sense. Unfortunately, this response with its lack of transparency placed Valerie in a vulnerable situation

with someone she did not know and did not trust. She ended up not hiring the person and looking elsewhere.

Transparency is important in most situations when we need to make decisions. Historically, transparency has not played a central role in healthcare because others, such as doctors, made most of our decisions for us. As individuals are asked to take on more responsibility both in care decisions as well as financial impact, transparency becomes more important. The rules and the players are clear. Normally, costs and contracts are disclosed as part of the decision- making process. This does not hold true for healthcare. People do not see healthcare as transactional. One's health is much more personal. In addition, there is lack of clear cost information. This creates a "shopability" challenge. In addition, payers are utilizing plan designs such as the use of high deductible health plans. The transition from co-pay to co-insurance have created greater out of pocket cost obligations to the consumer and have placed consumers in a situation where they are less insulated from the cost of care. The reality is that the system has placed consumers in a difficult situation. They are being asked to make thoughtful decisions without much of the available information. Most of us don't buy a car without using resources such as Consumer Reports or Edmunds to identify a reasonable cost and research the reliability of the car. That is exactly what is needed in healthcare and for the most part, with few exceptions, it is unavailable. Organizations such as GoodRx have brought cost information to consumers in an easy to understand and actionable manner. It has created a transparency tool that brings to the forefront the variation on price that exists associated with medications. An example of this is Famotidine, a medication used to treat and prevent ulcers. Through the use of GoodRx, a consumer would find that their out-of-pocket costs could range from $4 -$65 dollars for the same dose and quantity depending on where they purchase the medicine. More recently, Amazon has begun selling medications through a transparent cost model on their web site. As more tools become available to support transparency of costs, it will be up to the consumer as to whether they use these tools. A 2017 Health Affairs study showed that only 52% of consumers were aware of the cost of the care that they were receiving and only 12% utilized resources available to them to get a cost estimate. Consumer behavior will have to change if transparency tools are to become valuable.

It is not just consumers that articulate their frustration and confusion regarding costs and transparency. Infighting regarding costs is another area that creates distrust. None of the the stakeholders that we spoke with believed they should be responsible for creating or participating in cost transparency activities. The uniform response was that it was not their responsibility. When providers that we spoke to were asked about discussions with their patients in regard to cost, we got two major responses; "We have no idea what things cost. In fact, we know no more than our patients do about what things cost." "I don't trust the information even when we try to use cost estimates. They never seem to be right and then my patient comes back to me angry." One doctor that we spoke to stated "I went to medical school to understand illness and how to best treat it. I did not go to school to be a businessperson. If I wanted to go into business, I would have gotten my MBA. I am a healer and therefore went to medical school". A health plan executive stated, "cost is a conversation between the consumer and their doctor. This is not the Health plans role." In addition to perceived lack of responsibility, a number of additional barriers have been articulated. When asked why organizations are unwilling to offer transparency in cost information, organizations have stated that "it is too hard to produce", "it is confusing for the consumer", "disclosure of contractual agreement is not feasible" and "it will increase healthcare costs". When we talked to interviewees, they felt that these barriers to transparency created increased distrust. Statements such as "sounds like excuses to me" and "it felt like they were hiding something" were commonly articulated. Niall Brennan, the CEO of the Health Care Cost Institute speaks about the pushback being seen by hospital systems. He shared that the data is "frustratingly incomplete". He shares that it will take time to make it of use to consumers but at they should be able to begin to understand the variation of costs today. He uses the example of the cost of a c-section that varies in cost from $5,000-$50,000. (Liss, 2021) The reality is that we need to start somewhere. The data needs to become available in a usable form. Until that time, the lack of transparency will create challenges for consumers, and a "black eye" in trust for the rest of the industry.

America is at a moment of truth in regard to transparency and trust focused on healthcare costs. In addition to organizations such as GoodRx and Amazon who address the issue of price transparency, the United States government is also looking to address the issue of price transparency. The Healthcare Price Transparency Act requires that hospitals post rates for shoppable services in an easy to under-stand and actionable manner. In addition to the Healthcare Price Transparency Act, the government is also looking to address another transparency issue, that of surprise billing. As 2020 came to a close, Congress passed on a bipartisan basis a bill that would address sur-prise billing and reduce the burden on consumers that believed they were following the in- network provider process only to find that they were being billed hundreds if not thousands of dollars.

While the federal and state government are beginning to address issues on cost transparency, the words and actions of other stake-holder remain in conflict. Even with all stakeholders publicly agree-ing that the consumer should be featured at the center of the U.S. healthcare system, there is considerable pushback in regard to is-sues such as price transparency and surprise billing. Behind closed doors, many stakeholders are placing their own financial goals above that of the consumer. As hospital providers are working to put forth the legislated "shoppable services" in a transparent man-ner, some of these organizations are quietly increasing the costs of on those not addressed. This behavior has already infuriated some of the consumer advocacy organizations and has created a deeper crevice of distrust. There are a few outliers that have been more proactive and working to embrace cost transparency. One of those organizations, Baylor Scott & White began reaching out to their patients to provide them with a cost estimate of the services that they were scheduled to receive. In addition, they offer a cost estimator that gives the consumer a personalized cost that includes the consumer's benefits information as well as the health system's contracted rates. The organization hopes that this will improve the experience and relationship between the two stakeholders. It is not just consumers and providers that are confused by the lack of transparency in healthcare costs, a WoltersKluwer survey found 87% of hospital executives surveyed were also confused. The one thing that the American Medical Association and the insurance industry trade group, AHIP agree on is that they oppose recent legislation. This conflict of word and action is creating a trust dilemma with consumers. It is unclear as to what the final product of this legislation will look like. What is clear is that the issue of cost transparency will not disappear. It will be a moment of truth for stakeholders.

Transparency regarding quality, like price transparency can have a significant impact in healthcare. Consumers use a number of resources to research the quality of goods prior to making a purchase. It is part of the purchase process. It has become an expectation of consumers. It not only can increase trust in the provider but also for the healthcare industry as a whole. Unfortunately, getting that information is not easy. The McKinsey 2019 Consumer Health Insights Survey found that very few of consumers surveyed were able to find quality information such as outcomes, reputation, and experience, that would help them to make healthcare decisions. The most common sites that offer public reporting and that have been utilized are Healthgrades, ZocDoc, and the Consumer Assessment of Healthcare Providers and Systems (CAHPS), government websites such as Hospital Compare, Leapfrog and more recently sites such as Yelp and Angie's List. Consumers trust these third- party websites over those that are owned by Health Plans and Health Systems. They feel that sites owned by payers and other providers use quality transparency more as a marketing tool then as a reliable information source.

Although the public sites have brought value to consumers, they have created distrust and frustration in the provider community. Providers have articulated their concern over how quality and satisfaction are defined on these sites. In addition, they have voiced serious concerns over the accuracy of the measures. The online provider reviews are also grounds for many providers reduction in trust with their patients. A 2017 study published in the Journal of General Internal Medicine found that these online evaluations created a "strain" on the patient-provider relationship. (Holliday, 2017)

Quality transparency is not only important to the consumer but also to other healthcare entities. Entities such as the National Practitioner Data Bank (NPDB) have become an important tool for healthcare entities to have transparency into a physician's quality of care. The NPDB is a computer database run by the United States Department of Health and Human Services. It began in 1986 and including clinical privileges restrictions, actions against physicians' licenses, and medical malpractice awards. The Data Bank was created by Congress with the primary goals of improving health care quality, protecting the public and reducing health care fraud and abuse. Many physicians complain about the NPDB stating that the information is often misleading and is not actually transparent.

Transparency in healthcare should not only be focused on costs and quality. Transparency in action and motive are also factors in the health-care stakeholder trust equation. Like in other areas within American society, contractual agreements drive an individual's actions. What is often not considered is how that contractual action impacts other stake-holders. This is especially a cause for concern when the action can affect trust. Examples of this in the past have included "gag clauses" or the contractual obligation to withhold information between the patient and the provider. This has most often been seen when health plans contractually mandate that providers not share treatment options that are not covered by the insurance policy. For many years, these contracts were most common between physicians and their patients. More recently, these types of gag clause contractual language have extended to pharmacists and other providers. This type of contractual language creates widespread distrust due to perceived or real conflict of interest. Providers distrust the health plan for placing them in a position of withholding information to the patient and not fulfilling their obligation as healthcare providers. Patients distrust the provider and the health plan for putting financials ahead of their health. It places the patient in a position of asking, "who controls my care, my doctor or the insurance company." They feel that their doctor should always stand up for them.

Another area associated with contractual distrust is connected to pharmaceutical pricing. In order to understand the trust challenge associated with drug pricing one needs to understand that there are multiple stakeholders involved including the pharmaceutical manufacturer, health plan, employer, pharmacy benefits manager (PBM), retail pharmacy, wholesaler, and consumer. Each stakeholder has its own goals which are often in conflict with others. The most common and most controversial payment model includes a rebate. The rebate is a refund of a portion of the purchase price of the medication. These rebates are most commonly paid from the manufacturer to the PBM and then shared with either the health plan or the employer. Rebates are often used as a method to obtain preferential treatment by the PBM through formulary placement or through the impact of utilization management. Those that do not like the rebate model consider it a bribe or "pay for play" payment. There is also belief that the rebate model is not consumer friendly since it places greater cost on the shoulder of the consumer and creates a barrier to the consumer being able to get the safe and effective medication that will work best for them. Those that admire the rebate model state that the rebate has little impact on access to appropriate medicines and that it helps payers to underwrite healthcare costs. One consistent concern is the lack of transparency in the contractual arrangements associated with rebates. Many stakeholders within healthcare including providers, employers, and consumers, consider these "secret negotiations" that fly in the face of good healthcare.

Transparency's direct relationship to trust is not always the case. One study that focused on government decision making found that transparency did not create trust but in fact created confusion and distrust. There were assumptions that if the government was reporting information, bad behavior must be occurring. This led to a decrease in trust which was counter to the assumed outcome. (Triangale, 2019). Transparency around pharmaceutical payments to physicians for services rendered, is another example. When consumers were given transparent information about these payments, there was a reduction in trust. While some consumers and other healthcare stakeholders felt that providers being paid to speak, consult, or support cancer research trial was ethical and that it did not affect their trust in providers, others did not. Transparency in activities such as those identified in the Open Payments program have had a significant negative trust reset™. A 2019 Pew survey found that only 15% of consumers trusted that physicians were being transparent about conflicts of interest all of the time, 50% some of the time and 33% none of the time. (Pew, 2019) (Wheelock, 2020). Nevertheless, in most cases, transparency is the antidote to distrust. As Lucian Leape stated, "if transparency were a medication, it would be a blockbuster, with billions of dollars in sales and accolades the world over."

Recommendations

1.  Individual
    a.  Don't be afraid of transparency. In most cases, providers offer quality care.

    b. Know your data. The data associated with cost and quality are benchmarks that all individuals should be measuring themselves with.

    c. Individual providers should take cost and quality transparency seriously

    d. Individual providers should be transparent with their patients about their costs, their quality and any contractual arrangements that may directly impact their relationship with their patients and potential conflict of interest in delivering care.

2. Organizational

    a. Create a culture of the open sharing of information. This is a way to create public and consumer trust. This includes open communication between stakeholders both inside and external to the organization. Transparency requires a no-blame culture.

    b. Transparency needs to be recognized as an opportunity to differentiate yourself in the market.

    c. Create a continuous loop of information sharing and engagement with other stakeholders

    d. Create transparency tools simple to understand and actionable. Don't be afraid of honest and transparent information. Those that are difficult to understand, or use create negative trust resets™ can hurt the reputation of the organization.

    e. Understand that quality transparency tools can also help an organization and the associated individuals in their continuous quality activities.

# Conclusion

You can't go back and change the beginning, but you can
start where you are and change the ending.
C.S. Lewis

## WHY THIS BOOK IS IMPORTANT

This book is about trust. Trust as both an emotion and an action is
fundamental to the success of any society. It is often described as
the "glue of society". Trust is the central feature to all relationships
whether personal or professional as human connection is formed on
the basis of trust. It allows us to interact without fear. Over the last
twenty years we have seen societal trust in the United States deteriorating and we are now, as a country, in a trust crisis. The last four years
have created the greatest trust chasm since the civil war. This presents
huge challenges for our nation. The country is at a crossroad.

The country is not alone. Healthcare is also at a crossroad. Healthcare
as it exists today is not sustainable. While we are seeing great strides
in innovation, the United States struggles with access, quality and
cost of care. There is a great deal of experimentation occurring with
the hope of addressing these challenges. Many of these experiments
are focused on operational, organizational and financial transformation. It is our belief that while these issues are important, if we don't
address our significant trust issues, we will not get the outcomes that
we are hoping to achieve.

Healthcare does not exist in a vacuum. Secular trends and an overall paucity of trust within our country creates a challenging backdrop to trust across the healthcare ecosystem. These include decreased trust in institutions, significant polarization and partisanship creating distrust between friends, family and neighbors and the overarching societal focus on financial success at any cost. A 2020 Salesforce.com survey found

- 42% of individuals stated that they don't trust companies to tell the truth.
- 41% percent stated that they do not trust companies to act in society's or an individual's best interest as they focus on profit over people.
- 92% of organizations need to improve their trustworthiness.
- 61% stated that it is difficult to "earn my trust".

As we said above, trust is necessary in all aspects of our lives, but we need to ask if healthcare differs from other areas. The reality is that trust is foundational in healthcare. Consumer health is very personal. In fact, many would say that there is nothing as personal as our health. When our health is at risk, we become vulnerable. We need to know that those responsible for our health have our best interest in mind. Very few individuals feel that the healthcare system takes this responsibility seriously. Most of the stakeholders that we spoke to assumed that they were trusted. Some of this comes from a historical perspective when healthcare was based on a paternalistic system that deemed its "membership" to be respected and in some cases revered. These people were surprised when we shared some of the information that we collected, and they absorbed what people had to say. The few that understood the challenge that healthcare faces spoke of how they were trying to address the problem. Lacking trust within healthcare is the greatest barrier to improving our system, impacting both clinical outcomes and the increasing costs associated with health and healthcare in our country. We need to change the social contract between clinicians and society, clinicians and patients, clinicians and the healthcare system and across all stakeholders associated with healthcare. (Kornacki, JAMA)

We need to be clear that the challenges in trust across stakeholders in healthcare are not based solely on overall societal distrust. Change is unsettling but necessary. Throughout this book we discussed some of the factors that have created negative trust resets™ among stakeholders. The information in this book is collected from three sources, quantitative data that was collected by Julie and me, peoples' stories collected through interviews and information from third party resources.

Our research found four primary themes that need to be addressed if we are to succeed. The first rests on **relationships**. Over the last forty years, without our full realization, healthcare has transitioned from a relationship- based system to a financial based system. Along with this change, we have lost trust. Historically, the primary relationship in healthcare was between the physician and the patient. This was the bedrock of medicine. For the most part, this relationship no longer exists and where it does, it is often in flux. Longevity of relationship is a multiplier of trust. The system has dismantled it. The good news is that there are an increasing number of organizations such as Oak Street Health, Eden Health and Firefly that are working to create a new primary care provider team and consumer relationship. In speaking with these organizations, they articulate the need to re-build trust.

Although the primary care provider and consumer relationship is the cornerstone of trust in the clinical environment, there are additional relationships that are equally as important. It is not unusual for business decisions between healthcare organizations to be determined by procurement departments. Decisions are no longer made by evaluating capabilities or aligned goals. This creates an environment of commoditization and de-emphasizes trusting relationships. In order to create trust across the healthcare stakeholder spectrum we need to aim for "authentic relationships. People like to interact and work with people that they like and trust.

The second reoccurring theme is focused on the **healthcare system.** The definition of a system is "a set of things or actions that are organized, interconnected, thoughtful and coordinated to form a unified whole. (Oxford Dictionary) This is not what we have. To be successful, healthcare needs to be a team event with a focus on communication, collaboration and aligned goals. Similar to many other institutions, healthcare is not organized in a coordinated way that creates respect or trust across the system stakeholders. It is an institution that has knowledge and power at its base. Negotiations between organizations and individuals are based on a win-lose scenario. Incentives are often not aligned. Similar to the provider-consumer relationship, long term relationships rarely exist. We need to find ways to build consensus. This can only be done by identifying aligned goals and trying to understand the perspective of others.

In addition, the healthcare system has exchanged the term patient for the term **consumer**. Along with the renaming, they have placed new expectations on this individual. What has not occurred, is the creating of a system that supports these new expectations. Consumer expectations have changed over the last several years. They expect their experiences within the healthcare system to resemble those of other day to day activities. Experience, quality of service and affordable costs are table stakes. We talk about efficiency and effectiveness; we often do not talk about the experience. **Experience** has been found to be as important as the product or service that is being delivered with 76% of consumers stating that they are willing to change their providers if they do not like the experience. Interestingly, this has been found to be true for both business buyers and consumers. (Salesforce, 2020) One third of consumers said that they have chosen to forgo medical treatment because of their lack of trust in the care required. They state that this lack of trust is based on both their experience with the system and their fear that the system cares more about their own needs than the consumers. This is a frightening (WoltersKluwer Health July 2020)

Along with experience, profits and costs have created the most significant negative trust re-set™ for healthcare. When a healthcare organization achieves unicorn status it is headline news. You do not see the same type of media exposure for outstanding clinical outcomes. Both providers and consumers voiced their concerns of "profits over patients". Interestingly, we heard similar concerns from a number of non-clinical workers and executives. Almost everyone we spoke discussed how "the other guy" was profit driven and how that negatively impacted their organization. There is finger pointing between stakeholders with very few understanding the overall impact of healthcare financing. Most of those doing the finger pointing are doing little publicly to improve cost issues and therefore improve trust.

Most organizations do not realize the overarching impact that trust has on their success and **sustainability**. Over the last several years there has been an increased focus on sustainability for most organizations. Over 90% of S&P 500 organizations report on sustainability and corporate investors are requiring more focus on this element. Initially sustainability was equated with environmental issues. This is no longer the case. Consumer goods and services organizations such as Nike and healthcare organizations such as Cambia Health Solutions, have taken a much broader view of sustainability to include societal issues and long-term viability alongside of environmental issues as part of their sustainability assessments and programs. Unfortunately, many of these organizations have yet to understand the correlation between trust and corporate sustainability. "To earn trust, money and power aren't enough; you have to show concern for others. You cannot buy trust in the supermarket. (The Dali Lama). It is time for organizations to increase the focus on trust as a determinant to future success and sustainability. Just as many organizations utilize net promoter scores as a longitudinal metric, they need to begin to implement trust assessments on the same basis and report it as part of their sustainability programs. Trust is a muscle that we all have to develop and maintain if we hope to succeed. Actions leading to trust are not a cost but an investment.

The path to reset trust in the American Healthcare system does not have to be overwhelming. Healthcare can no longer be a blood sport. We cannot just wish for it; we must demand it from ourselves and others. A band of sisters and brothers leading with trust. There is no one person to blame, we are all to blame. In many cases, we are unaware of the impact of our actions. Whether it be a clinician that does not understand the importance of building a strong relationship with their patients, a physician that is not acting as a team- mate with other members of the team, a consumer that is not being honest with their healthcare provider, a pharmaceutical manufacturer that rewards their employees for selling medications that may not be appropriate for the consumer, or a payer or service provider that has placed profit above care; we all need to engage in this effort.

Every stakeholder directly involved in healthcare and others that indirectly involved, such as the media, have played a role in the degradation of trust that has occurred. That means that we all have to play a role in re-engaging in trust. "There's a lot in healthcare that could be vastly improved, and those are the little things"(Hayley Hovious, President of Nashville Health Care Council). As Hayley states, small changes can make a big difference. The research on trust leads us to the same conclusion. We propose that each individual look to the acronym CAARE ™ as a benchmark to beginning to make small changes.

**C**ommunication
**A**ttitude
**A**ssessment
**R**elationship
**E**xperience

The regaining of trust will not be easy and will take time. All stakeholders will have to be honest and make a concerted effort if we hope to move the needle in the trust meter. Actions will have to change. No one segment of healthcare can rebuild trust on its own. If we all believe that trust is necessary to achieve the desired and necessary goals, we will have to step outside our traditional behaviors, actions and activities and move to a new norm. This is the only way that we will regain the trust necessary to achieve. It will take all of us. I challenge each of you reading this book to find one behavior or action that you can take to help us regain trust. Not only will we be better off as a healthcare system and a country but each of us will be better off. None of us can take trust for granted. One cannot assume that if you are trusted today that you will be trusted in the future. Those that are deeply trusted today do have a better chance of retaining trust in the future. Improving trust can feel overwhelming. There are some things that we can't control. We need to choose whether to be an "bystander or an upstander". Re-engaging in trust will require a number of changes both structural and in mind set. We cannot do this without focus and motivation. Some of these changes need to be done at an individual level and others at a systemic level. We need to take one step at a time. Some people that read this book will come away frustrated and potentially even angry. Others that read this book will come away energized because they see that a path for all to re-engage in trust. As an idealistic pragmatist, my hope is that each person that reads this book can find one action that can build on trust and how they can be part of the solution. We all need a highly functional healthcare system. We have to remember, "we are not enemies". We all learn to trust. We actually yearn for trust and thrive on it. Frustration can pull at the threads of trust. This can be addressed. I hope that the "better angels of our nature" bring us together in the battle to re-engage in trust. (Abraham Lincoln, 1861)

# Health Intelligence
# Partners Trust Survey

1.  What is your age?
2.  Do you or any family member work in healthcare?
3.  How would you describe your gender?
4.  How do you describe yourself? (race/ethnicity)
5.  On a scale of 1 - 10 (with 1 meaning great and 10 meaning poor), how would you describe your health?
6.  Do you have any chronic or long-term medical problems (for example, like asthma, heart disease or diabetes)? If yes, how many?
7.  Has your doctor prescribed a medicine for you to take daily or weekly? If yes, how do you take them
8.  Do you take vitamins, minerals, supplements, or other homeopathic treatments?
9.  Do you have a primary care doctor (i.e., doctor you see for regular check-ups and for non-emergency care)? If no, where do you go?
10. How often do you see or talk to your primary care doctor?
11. Do you trust your doctor? If yes, what makes you trust your doctor? If no, what makes you NOT trust your doctor?
12. Are you comfortable talking to your doctor?
13. Do you believe that your doctor does what is best for you?
14. How long have you been going to this doctor?

15. If you don't understand your doctor's instructions or explanations, do you ask them to explain or ask them questions? If no, why?
16. For healthcare treatment/advice do you trust any of the following? (check all that apply)
17. Do you see other healthcare professionals besides your doctor? (check all that apply)
18. Since you see these other health professionals, do you trust him or her?
19. Have you gotten any of the following tests (preventive) in the past year? (check all that apply)
20. If you have NOT gotten any of these tests, why? (check all that apply)
21. Do you track your activity (eating, sleeping or walking)?
22. If you gave someone information about your health or illnesses, who would you trust it with? (check all that apply)
23. Healthcare has been in the news a great deal over the last few
24. years. How well do you understand the healthcare system, insurance, and how it can help you?
25. Thinking about your experiences, do you trust the healthcare system?
26. Since the election would you say that you trust the healthcare system?
27. Since the election would you say that you trust your doctor?
28. Since the election would you say that you trust your friends and neighbors?

# References

1.  2019 Digital Health Consumer Survey. Accenture. February 2019
2.  2019 Healthcare Consumer Trends Report. NRC Health
3.  Abbas R. Carroll N. et al. Trust Factors in Healthcare Technology: A Healthcare Professional Prospective. 11th International Conference on Health Informatics. January 2018
4.  Accenture 2019 Digital Health Consumer Survey. Today's Consumers Reveal the Future of Healthcare. Accenture Consulting
5.  Accenture. Elevating the Patient Experience to Fuel Growth. Accenture Consumer Health Experience Survey 2020.
6.  Arora VM. et al. Why Bolstering Trust in Journalism Could Help Strengthen Trust in Medicine. June 11, 2019; 321(22): 2159-60
7.  Arpey N. Gaglioti A. et al. How Socio-economic Status Effects Patients Perception of Healthcare. Journal of Primary Care & Community Health. 2017; 8(3):169-173
8.  Arterburn D. Wellman R. et al. Introducing Decision Aids at Group Health was Linked to Sharply Lower Hip and Knee Surgeries and Costs. Health Affairs. 2012; 31(9):2094-2104
9.  Ashton CM. Haider P. et al. Racial and ethnic disparities in the use of Health services: Bias, preference or poor communication? Journal of General Internal Medicine. 2003; 18:146-152

10. Babaian J. Importance of Trust in Healthcare. Healthcare Leadership Blog. January 23, 2018; #Hcldr

11. Bachai S. Black Americans Don't Trust Our Healthcare System-Here's Why. The Hill. August 24, 2017; http://the-hill.com/blogs/pundits-blog/healthcare/347780-black-americans-don't-have-trusts-in-our-healthcare-system

12. Baden L. Solomon C. et al. The FDA and the Importance of Trust. NEJM. September 30, 2020.

13. Baker D., Trust in Healthcare in the Time of Covid-19. JAMA. December 15,2020.324(23); 2373-2375

14. Bandura A. Guide for Constructing Self Efficacy Scales, Self Efficacy Beliefs in Adolescents. 2006: 307-337

15. Barlas S. Employers and Drugstores Press for PBM Transparency. Pharmacy & Therapeutics. March 2015; 40(3):206-208

16. Bauchner H. Trust in Healthcare. JAMA. Feb 12, 2019; 321(6):547

17. Baruah B. 'The Importance of Trust in Healthcare | LinkedIn' Linkedin.com, January 5, 2017; https://www.linkedin.com/pulse/importance-trust-healthcare-biswajit-dutta-baruah/

18. Baird, K. Trust at the Core of the Patient Experience. Becker's Hospital Review. May 6, 2013.

19. Benjamins M. Religious Influences on Trust in Physicians and the Healthcare System. International Journal of Psychiatry in Medicine. 2006; 36(1):69-83

20. Berger J. Medical Liability for Pediatricians. 2004

21. Berger J. McAbee G. Deitschel C. Pediatric Medicolegal Education in the 21st Century. Pediatrics. 2006;117(5):1790-1792

22. Berkowitz E. Medicare and Medicaid; The Past as Prologue. Health Care Financial Review. Spring 2008; 29(3)

23. Birkhauer J. et al. "Trust in the HealthCare Professional and Health Outcome: A Meta-Analysis". PLOS ONE. February

7, 2017; *12*(2): e0170988 https://doi.org/10.1271/journal.pone.0170988

24. Blair R. Morse B. Tsai L. Public Health and Public Trust. Social Science and Medicine. Jan 2017; 172:89-97

25. Blendon R. Public Health: Matters of Trust Symposium. Harvard University of Public Health. 2002

26. Blendon R. et al. "Public Trust in Physicians-U.S. Medicine in International Perspective. NEJM. October 23, 2014; 371(17): 570-572

27. Blendon R. et al. Public Trust in Physicians. NEJM. 2014; 37(17):1570-1572

28. Berwick, D. Politics and Healthcare. JAMA. October 9, 2018

29. Borah P. Media Effect Theory. January 4, 2016; https://doi.org/10.1002/9781118541555.wbiepc156

30. Brenan M. Americans Trust in Mass Media Edges Down to 41%. Politics. September 26, 2019

31. Boulware L.E. et al. "Race and Trust in the Health Care System." *Public Health Reports*. 2003; 118(4): 358 –365

32. Boyle J. Brassell T. Dayton J. As cases increase, Americans trust in COVID 19 information from federal, state, and local governments continue to decline. ICF Insights in Health. July 20, 2020

33. Brooks, D. America is Having a Moral Convulsion. The Atlantic. October 5, 2020.

34. Brown T. Bussell J. Dutta S. Davis K. Strong S. Mathew S. Medication Adherence: Truth and Consequences. American Journal of the Medical Sciences. April 2016; 351(4):387-399

35. Buchan N. Croson R. et al. Trust and Gender: An Examination of Behavior and Beliefs in the Investment Game. Journal of Economic Behavior & Organization. 68. 2008: 466-476

36. Bulik B. Pharma's Reputation Has Soared during Covid 19 pandemic. FiercePharma. April 21, 2020

37. Caterinicchio RP. Testing Plausible Path Models of Interpersonal Trust in Patient-Physician Treatment

Relationships. Social Science in Medicine. 13(1), 1979: 81 –99

38. Chambers JD. Panzer AD. et al. Little consistency in evidence cited by commercial plans for specialty drug coverage. Health Affairs. 2019; 38(11): 1882-1886

39. Chwistek M. "Are You Wearing Your White Coat?" Telemedicine in the Time of Pandemic. JAMA. July 14, 2020; 324(2):149-150

40. Collado, M. Oakman T. Shah M. To Improve Health Care, How Do We Build Trust and Respect for Patients. Health Affairs. September 26, 2917.

41. Collins KS. Hughs DL. Doty M. Diverse Communities, Common Concerns. Commonwealth Fund 2001 Healthcare Quality Survey: 30,33

42. Coppins M. The Man Who Broke Politics. The Atlantic. November 2018.

43. Corbie-Smith G, Thomas SB. et al. Distrust, Race and Research, Archives of Internal Medicine 2002; 162(21): 2958-63

44. Coronovirus Disease 2019, Trust, Facts and Democracy. Trust in Institutions. Pew Research Center

45. Crawshaw R. Rogers D. et al. Patient-Physician Covenant. JAMA. May 17, 1995; 273(19)

46. Crnkovich P. Clarin D. How Millennials Are Reshaping Healthcare's Future, Kaufman Hall. 2019

47. Curlin F. Roach BS. Gorawara-Batt R. When Patients Choose Faith over Medicine. Archives of Internal Medicine. 2005; (165): 88-91

48. Dalen J. Waterbrook K. Alpert J. Why do so Many Americans Oppose the Affordable Care Act? The American Journal of Medicine. August 2015; 128(8):807-810

49. Dalen J. Where Have the Generalists Gone? The American Journal of Medicine. July 2017; 130(7)

50. Davis J. Building Trust. TEDX USA. December 6, 2014

51. De Law N. Medicare: 35 Years of Service. Health Care Financing Review. Fall 2000; 22(1): 75-103.

52. DeLombaerde G. "Revive Health Study: Trust in Health Care System Declining." Nashville Post. September 25, 2017; https://nashvillepost.com/business/health-care/article/20976737/revivehealth-study-trust-in-health-care-stystem-still-declining

53. DePaulo B. Kashy D. et al. Lying in Everyday life. Journal of Personality and Social Psychology. 1996. 70(5):979-995.

54. Dodge J. Pharmacy Benefit Managers and Their Role in Drug Spending. Commonwealth Fund. April 22, 2019; (https://doi.org/10.26099/njmh-en20)

55. Drettwan J. Kjos A. An Ethical Analysis of Pharmacy Benefit Manager Practices. Pharmacy. June 2019; 7(2):65 (doi.3390/pharmacy7020065)

56. Edwin AK. Don't Lie but Don't Tell the Whole Truth: The Therapeutic Privilege-Is it Ever Justified. Ghana Medical Journal. 2008 Dec; 42(4):156-161.

57. Eisen S. Davos. 2017; http://www.weforum.org. assessed 6/12/2019

58. Enabnit A. Do you Lie to Your Doctor? TermLife2Go.com. February 20, 2020

59. Flannigan N. National Healthcare Trust Index- Healthcare Dive. October 26, 2015.

60. Frankel RM. Tilden VP. Suchman A. Physicians Trust in One Another. JAMA. 2019; 321(14):1345-1346

61. Frosch D. Tai-Seale. M. Respect-What it Means to Patients. Journal of General Internal Medicine. 2014 March; 29(3).; 427-428

62. Funk C. Kennedy B. Hefferon M. Vast Majority of Americans Say Benefits of Childhood Vaccines Outweigh Risks. Pew Research Center. February 2, 2017

63. Funk C. et al. Trust and Mistrust in Americans' View of Scientific Experts. Pew Research Center 2019 study. August 2, 2019.

64. Fukuyama F. Trust: The Social Virtues and the Creation of Prosperity. New York, Free Press

65. Furumo K. Pearson J. Gender-Based Communication Styles, Trust, and Satisfaction in Virtual Teams. Journal of Information, Information Technology and Organizations. 2007; (2):47-60

66. Gallup Polls. State of the Workplace. 2013

67. Gallup Polls. 2013; Https://www.gallup.com/poll/1654/honesty-ethics-professions.aspx

68. Gallup Polls. Honesty, Trust and Integrity Survey. 2019; www.gallup.com

69. Ganguli I. Zhou S. et al. Declining Use of Primary Care Among Commercially Insured Adults in the United States. 2008-2016. Annals of Internal Medicine. February 4, 2020.

70. Guerrero N. Mendes de Leon C. et al. Soc. Determinants of Trust in Health Care in an Older Population. Journal of Geriatrics. March 2015; 63(3):553-557.

71. Giddens. Consequences of Modernity. Policy Press. 1991

72. Girgis L. Why Doctors are Losing the Public's Trust. Physicians Weekly.com Blog. December 18, 2017

73. Giuliani S. Will Organizations trust health care organizations after COVID 19? Deloitte Blog. May 5, 2020

74. Grande D. Shea J. Armstrong K. J General Internal Medicine. Pharmaceutical industry gifts to physicians; patient beliefs and trust in physicians and the healthcare system. 2012; 27(3):274-279

75. Gray B. Trust and Trustworthy Care in the Managed Care Era. Health Affairs. 16(1)

76. Gray J. Men are From Mars, Women are From Venus. HarperCollins Publishing. 1992

77. Green M. Masters R. James B. et al. Do Gifts from the Pharmaceutical Industry Affect Trust in Physicians? Family Medicine. 2012; 44(5):325-31

78. Grob R. Darien G. Meyers D. Why physicians should trust in patients. JAMA. 2019; 321(14):1347-1348

79. Gruber L. Shadle M. and Polich C. From Movement to Industry: The Growth of the HMOs. Health Affairs. Summer 1988; 7(3)

80. Gupta A. Physician verses non-physician CEO: The effect of a leader's professional background on the quality of hospital management and healthcare. Journal of Hospital Administration. July 2019; 8(5):47-51

81. Gupta R. Binder L. Rebuilding Trust and Relationships in Medical Centers. JAMA. December 15, 2020. 324(23). 2361-2362.

82. Haas BW. Ishak A. Anderson I. Filkowski M. The Tendency to Trust is Reflected in Human Brain Structure. Neuroimage. February 15, 2015; (107):175-181

83. Hagland M. "OK, Boomers": Will Millennials and Gen Z Young People Turn the Tables on Baby Boom Healthcare Leaders. Healthcare Innovation. December 27, 2019.

84. Hall M.A. et al, "Measuring Patients' Trust in Their Primary Care Providers." Medical Care Research. 2002; 59 (3): 293 –318.

85. Hamel L. Kearney A. The KFF Health Tracking Poll. Kaiser Family Foundation. September 10, 2020

86. Harris Poll. Harris Poll Study of Reputation Equity and Risk Across Healthcare Sector. 2016

87. Harvard Business Review. June 2009

88. Healthcare 2001: A Strategic Assessment of the Healthcare Environment in the United States. AHA. 2002

89. Heath S. As Health IT Evolves, Patient Provider Trust Remains Essential. PatientEngagementHIT, December 10, 2018.

90. Heath S. Patient-Provider Communication Falls Short of Patient Expectation. November 11, 2018

91. Heller K. Washington Post. December 24, 2019

92. Hertling M. Growing Physician Leaders. Rosetta Books. May 2016

93. Holdsworth L. et al., Beyond Satisfaction Scores: Exploring Emotionally Adverse Patient Experiences. American Journal of Managed Care. May 2019: 212

94. Holland, K. Fighting with your spouse? Its probably about this. CNBC. February 4, 2015.

95. Holliday A. Kachalia A. et al. Physician and Patient Views on Public Physician Rating Websites: A Cross-Sectional Study. Journal of Internal Medicine 2017. 32; 626-631.

96. Huesch M. Mosher T. Using it or Losing It? NEJM. May 4, 2017

97. Jain S. Lucey C. The Enduring Importance of Trust in the Leadership of Health Care Organizations. JAMA. December 15, 2020. 324(23):2363-2364.

98. Jellinek M. Erosion of Patient Trust in Large Medical Centers. Hastings Center Report. June 1976: 16-17

99. Johnston SC. The Risk and Cos of Limited Clinician and Patient Accountability in Healthcare. JAMA. Published online September 30, 2019; doi:10.1001/jama.2019.14832

100. Jones B. Increasing share of Americans favor a single government program to provide health care coverage. Pew Research Center. August 2020

101. Katz J. The Silent World of Doctor and Patient. JHU Press. 2002

102. Kao A.C. et al. "The Relationship between Method of Physician Payment and Patient Trust." Journal of the American Medical Association. *1998; 280* (19): 1708 –1714

103. Keckley P. "The Trust Chasm in Health Care: Analysis of the 2016 Trust Survey." November 2, 2016; https://hhnmag.com/articles/7802-the-trust-chasm-in-healthcare-analysis-of-the-2016-trust-survey.

104. Khuller D. Do You Trust the Medical Profession? The New York Times. January 23, 2018. The Upshot. https:www.nyt.com/2018/01/23/upshot/do-you-trust

105. Khullar D. Building Trust in Healthcare-Why, Where and How. JAMA. August 13,2019; 322(6):507-509

106. Khullar D. Patient Consumerism, Health Relationships and Rebuilding Trust in Healthcare. JAMA. December 15, 2020. 324(23). 2359-2360

107. King William. Examining African Americans Mistrust of the Health Care System: Expanding the Research Question. Public Health Reports. July-August 2003; 118:366-367

108. Knapp K. Ray M. et al. The Role of Community Pharmacies in Diabetes Care. July 2005

109. Kocher R. Emmanuel Z. Will Robots Replace Doctors? Brookings. March 5, 2019

110. Kornacki MJ. Silverman J. Chokshi. From Distrust to Building Trust in Clinician-Organization Relationships. JAMA. May 14 2019; 321(8): 1761-1762

111. Kraetschmer N. Sharpe N. et al. How does trust affect patient preferences for participation in decision making? Health Expectations. 2004:317-326

112. Kramer R. Tyler T. Trust in Organizations: Frontiers in Theory and Research, Thousand Oakes, CA. Sage Publications 1996 Pearson SD, et al. Patients Trust in physicians. 2000; 15(7):509-513

113. Kruse K. "What is Employee Engagement" Forbes. June 22, 2012

114. Kurtz SF. "The Law of Informed Consent: From Doctor is Right to Patient has Rights." Syracuse Law Review. 2000; 50(4):1243-1260

115. Lee J. Sniderman B. Marquard B. Embedding trust into COVID 19 recovery. Deloitte Insights. April 23, 2020

116. Lee J. Kang K. et al. Associations Between COVID 19 Misinformation Exposure and Belief with COVID 19 Knowledge and Preventative Behaviors. Journal of Medical Internet Research. November 2020; 22.

117. Lee T. et al. A Framework for Increasing Trust Between Patients and the Organizations That Care for Them. JAMA. Feb 12, 2019; 321(6):539-540

118. Lee PV. Berwick D. Sinsky CA. Building trust between the government and clinicians; person to person and organization to organization. JAMA. 2019; 321(18):1763-1764

119. Levinson W. Physician-Patient Communication. A Key to Malpractice Prevention. JAMA. 1994;272(20):1619-1620

120. Lewicki R. Tomlinson E. Gillespie N. Models of Interpersonal Trust Development; Theoretical Approaches, Empirical Evidence and Future Directions. Journal of Management. December 2006; 32(6):991-1022

121. Liu H. Fang H. Rizzo J. HMO and Patient Trust in Physicians: A longitudinal Study. International Journal of Applied Economics. March 2013; 10910:1-21.

122. Liss S. CMS audits small slice of hospitals for price transparency, probes complaints. Healthcare Dive. January 11, 2021

123. Lowry F. Costs of Breast Cancer Surgery Can Be Financial Burden. August 8, 2019

124. Macrae C. Uncles M. Rethinking Brand Management. Journal of Product and Brand Management. University of New South Wales. 1997:64-77

125. Martens G. Gerritsen L. et al. Fear of the coronavirus: Predictors in an online study conducted in March 2020. Journal of Anxiety Disorders. 2020; 74:1-8.

126. Mathews K. Meeting the Demands of the Younger Patient, Medical Economics. June 25, 2019:31

127. McCarthy J. Seven in 10 Maintain Negative View of U.S. Healthcare System. Wellbeing. January 14, 2018

128. McPhillips D. Majority of Americans Don't Trust Government with their Health. U.S. News and World Report. March 26, 2020

129. Mechanic D. Schlesinger M. "The Impact of Managed Care on Patients' Trust in Medical Care and Their Physicians. Journal of the American Medical Association. *1996; 275*(21):1693 –1697

130. Michael M.L. Business Ethics. The Law of Rules. Working Paper No. 19. March 2006

131. Levinsky NG. The Doctor's Master. NEJM. 1984; 311:1573-1575

132. Medical Economics. How Implicit bias harms patient care. June 10, 2019:4

133. Meeting the Demands of the Younger Patient. Medical Economics. June 25,2019:31,

134. Merriam-Webster Dictionary. www.merraim-webster.com. Accessed March 30, 2109 Oxford Dictionary, Accessed March 30, 2019.

135. Mewes J. Giordano G. Self-raging health, generalized trust, and the Affordable Care Act. Social Science and Medicine. 190:48-56

136. Moments of Truth. Alegeus Healthcare. 2016

137. Montgomery T, Berns J. et al. Transparency as a Trust Building Practice in Physicians Relationships with Patients. JAMA. December 15, 2020. 324(23): 2365-2366.

138. Morgan J. The Decline of Trust in the United States. May 20, 2014. Doi; https://medium.com/@monarchjogs/the-decline-of-trust-in-the-united-states-fb8ab719b82a

139. Moscovitch B. Americans Want Federal Government to Make Sharing Electronic Health Data Easier. Pew Research. September 20, 2020

140. Toward Better Value. National Pharmaceutical Council. 2017

141. Nasher J. Convinced: How to Prove Your Competence and Win People Over. 2018.

142. NRC Healthcare Consumer Trend Report. January 2019

143. O'Brien B. Do you See What I See? Reflections on the Relationship Between Transparency and Trust. Academic Medicine. June 2019; 94(6)

144. O'Brien J. Chantler C. Confidentiality and the duties of care. Journal of Medical Ethics. 2003; 29(1)).

145. Ojeda C. The Effect of 9/11 on the Heritability of Political Trust. Political Psychology. February 1, 2016; 37(1):73-78

146. Oliver Wyman Survey. 2018

147. Ortiz-Ospina E. Roser M. Trust. OurWorldInData.org. May 2020

148. Ozawa S. The Role of Trust in Health Care Settings: Does Trust Matter. Oxford Policy Institute. June 2008.

149. Ozawa, S. et al. How do you measure trust in the health system? A systematic review of the literature. Social Science & Medicine. August 2013; 91:10-13

150. Panetta G. These 9 political friendships proved party lines don't have to divide Americans. Business Insider. November 15, 2018

151. Peek M, et al., Patient Trust in Physicians and Shared Decision Making Among African Americans with Diabetes. Health Communications. 2013; 28(6):616-623

152. Penman D.T. et al. Informed Consent for Investigational Chemotherapy: Patients' and Physicians' Perceptions. Journal of Clinical Oncology 1984; 2(7): 849 –855.

153. Perez SL. Weissman A. et al, US Internists perspectives on discussing cost of care with patients. Annals of Internal Medicine. 2019; 170:539-455

154. Pew Research Center, Public sees science and technology as net positives for society. July 26, 2016.

155. Pollitz K. Rae M. et al. An examination of surprise medical bills and proposals to protect consumers from them. KFF. February 2020.

156. Poulin M. Haase C. Growing to Trust: Evidence that Trust Increases and Sustains Well-Being Across the Life Span.

Social Psychology and Personality Science. March 2, 2015; 6(6): 614-621

157. Rainie L. Keeter S. Perrin A. Trust and Distrust in America. U.S. Politics and Policy. Pew Research Center. July 22, 2019

158. Ramsey Solutions; Financial Education and Success Company.

159. Reeve J. The Four C's of Rebuilding Trust in Health Care. October 29, 2014; https://healthinsight.org/about-us/healthinsight-blog/entry/1-healthinsight-blog/63-the-four-c's-of-rebuilding-trust-in-heath-care.

160. Rikhi R. Transparency of Medication Costs: A Method of Building Patient Trust. Academic Medicine. May 2019; 949(5)

161. Romano, P. Understanding Consumers Views of Cost Sharing, Quality and Network Choice. AcademyHealth.. March 2019.

162. Rose A. Peters N. Shea JA. et al. Development and testing of the health care system distrust scale. J General Internal Medicine. 2004; 19(1): 57-63

163. Roter D. The Patient-Physician Relationship and its Implications for Malpractice Litigation. Journal of Health Care Law Policy. 2006;(9):311

164. Rowe R. Calnan M. Trust Relations in Healthcare- the New Agenda. European Journal of Public health. 2006; 16(1)

165. Safran D.G. et al. Linking Primary Care Performance to Outcomes of Care. Journal of Family Practice. 1998; 47(3):213-220

166. Safran D.G. et al. Switching Doctors: Predictors of Voluntary Disenrollment from a Primary Physician's Practice. *Journal of Family Practice*. 2001; 50(2):130-136

167. Salesforce.com. State of the Connected Customer. 2020

168. Sandy LG. Pham HH. Levine S. Building trust between physicians, hospitals, payers: A renewed opportunity for transforming US healthcare. JAMA. 2019; 321(10): 933-934

169. Schleifer D. Consumer Valuation of Providers, Services and Venues in Three Complex Care Situations. AcademyHealth. July 2017.

170. Schultz A. Top Barriers to Participation in Clinical Trials. Forte Health. October 12, 2017

171. Schwartz J. Early History of Prepaid Medical Care Plans. Bulletin of the History of Medicine. Sept.-October 1965; 39(5): 450-476.

172. Seckin G. Health Information on the Web and Consumers Perspective on Health Professionals' Responses to Information Exchange. Medicine 2.0 2014. July-December; 3)2)

173. Shaw G. Patients don't trust health information technology. Fierce Healthcare. January 5, 2017

174. Shore D. The Trust Crisis in Healthcare. Oxford Press. 2007

175. Shore D. The Trust Prescription for Healthcare. 2012

176. Shrank W. Rogstad T, et al. Waste in the US Health Care System. JAMA. 2019;322(15):1501-1509.

177. Shryock T. Replacing Doctors. Medical Economics. January 30, 2019

178. Sinek S. Start with Why. 2009.

179. Sinek S, Why Differentiate Acquaintances from Friends. TEDx. April 6, 2011,

180. Singh O, Phillips K et al. Eliciting the patient's agenda. J General Internal Medicine. 2019. 34(1); 36-40

181. Singh P. Campbell T. et al. Development of a Culturally Tailored Motivational Interviewing Based Intervention to Improve Medication Adherence in South Asian Patients. Patient Preference and Adherence. 2020; 14:757-765

182. Singleton M. Can We Trust Government with our Medical Care? Association of American Physicians and Surgeons. June 8, 2019.

183. Sisk B. Frankel R. et al. The Truth about Truth Telling in American Medicine: A Brief History. The Permanente Journal. 2016 Summer. 20(3): 74-77.

184. Sklar DP. Trust is a two-way street. Academy Medicine. 2016; 91(2):155-158

185. Starr P. The Social Transformation of American Medicine. 2nd ed. New York. Basic Books Inc. 2017

186. Stevens R. Health Care in the Early 1960s. Health Care Finance Review. 1996; 18(2)

187. Sun E. Mello M. et al. Assessment of Out of Network Billing for Privately Insured Patients Receiving Care in In Network Hospitals. JAMA Internal Medicine. 2019; 179(11):1543-1550.

188. Tedeschi, B. 6 in 10 doctors report abusive remarks from patients: Patient prejudice Survey. STAT. October 18, 2017

189. Ten Ways to Rebuild Trust in Media and Democracy. Aspen Institute Communications and Society Program. February 5. 2019.

190. TermLife2Go.com. February 24, 2020

191. The Physician Charter on medical professionalism. ABIM 2002; https://abimfoundation.org/what-we-do/physician-charter.

192. Thom D.H. et al. Patient-Physician Trust." Journal of Family Medicine. 1997; 44(2)

193. Thom D.H. et al. Validation of a Measure of Patients' Trust in Their Physician: The Trust in Physician Scale. *Medical Care*. 1999; 137(5):510-517

194. Thom D.H. Hall. M.A. and Pawlson G. "Measuring Patients' Trust in Physicians When Assessing Quality of Care." Health Affairs. July1,2004; 23(4):124-132 https://doi.org/10.1277/hlthaff.23.4.124

195. Thorne S.E. Robinson C.A. "Reciprocal Trust in Health Care Relationships." *Journal of Advanced Nursing*. 1988; 13(6):782-789

196. Traugott M. Brader T. et al. How Americans Responded: A Study of Public Reactions.Doi:https://citeseerx.ist.psu.edu/viewdoc/download?doi=10.1.1.526.5976&rep=rep1&type=pdf)

197. Tringale, K. Hattangadi-Guth J. Truth, Trust and Transparency-The Highly Complex Nature of Patients Perceptions of Conflicts of Interest in Medicine. JAMA. April 12, 2019; 2(4)

198. Truog R. "Evolution of a Relationship." New England Journal of Medicine. August 2012; 366(7)

199. Trust and Communication in Healthcare: Key Findings | The Trust Project. The Trust Project at Northwestern University. Accessed Jan 23, 2018. https://www.kellog.northwestern.edu/trust-project.Trust, Facts and Democracy 2019. Pew Research Center

200. Trust in Healthcare Undermined by 'Bad Apples', New Research Reveals." ScienceDaily. November 3, 2017; https://www.sciencedaily.com/releases/2017/11/171103085701.htm.

201. Throw J. Gans R. As Seen on TV: Health Policy Issues in TV Medical Dramas. Kaiser Family Foundation. July 2002.

202. Ventola C. Social Media and Health Care Professionals: Benefits, Risks, and Best Practices. P & T Journal. July 2014; 39(7): 491-499.

203. Verghese A. Hard Cures; Doctors themselves could take several steps to reduce malpractice suits. New York Times. March 16, 2003

204. Walker T. Five Things that Consumers Want from Healthcare. Managed Care Executive. November 24, 2019.

205. Wesson D. Lucey C. Cooper L. Building Trust in Health Systems to Eliminate Health Disparities. JAMA. 322(2):111-112

206. Wheelock A. Bechtel C. et al. Human Centered Design and Trust in Medicine. JAMA. December 15, 2020. 324(23); 2369-2370.

207. Who do you trust when it comes to your business? September 26, 2019

208. Yachitz A. et al. Misrepresentation of Randomized Controlled Trials in Press Releases and News Coverage. PLOS Med. 2012; 9(9)

209. Yao C. Kulber D. Patients Can't Afford for Doctors to Misunderstand the Healthcare Business. January 22, 2020; www.qz.com

210. Yeung E. Pharmacists Becoming Physicians: For Better or Worse? Pharmacy. September 2018; 6(3):71 (doi: 10.3390/pharmacy6030071

211. Young W. Koning A. et al. Health Information Seeking and Trust in Sources. The "Health Matters Poll" Series. Rutgers Eagleton Center for Public Interest Polling. February 2020.

212. Zac P. How Our Brains Decide When to Trust. Harvard Business Review Ascend. July 18, 2019

213. Zac P. The Neuroscience of Trust. Harvard Business Review. January-February 2017.

214. Ziegler MG. Lew P. Singer BC. The accuracy of drug information from pharmaceutical sales representatives. JAMA. 1995; 273:1296-98

215. Zolkefli Y. The Ethics of Truth Telling in Healthcare Settings. Malaysian Journal of Medical Sciences. 2018 May; 25(3): 135-139.

CPSIA information can be obtained
at www.ICGtesting.com
Printed in the USA
LVHW030116070921
697109LV00002B/9